The Inner Cause

A Psychology of Symptoms from A to Z

The Inner Cause

A Psychology of Symptoms from A to Z

Martin Brofman

𝆑 FINDHORN PRESS

Findhorn Press
One Park Street
Rochester, Vermont 05767
www.findhornpress.com

Findhorn Press is a division of Inner Traditions International

Disclaimer

The information in this book is given in good faith and is neither intended to diagnose any physical or mental condition nor to serve as a substitute for informed medical advice or care. Please contact your health professional for medical advice and treatment. Neither author nor publisher can be held liable by any person for any loss or damage whatsoever which may arise from the use of this book or any of the information therein.

Library of Congress Cataloging-in-Publication Data

Names: Brofman, Martin, author.
Title: The inner cause : a psychology of symptoms from A to Z / Martin
  Brofman.
Description: Rochester, Vermont : Findhorn Press, [2018] | Includes
  bibliographical references and index.
Identifiers: LCCN 2018017232 (print) | LCCN 2018017748 (e-book) |
  ISBN 9781844097531 (paperback) | ISBN 9781844097593 (e-book)
Subjects: LCSH: Mind and body therapies. | Healing. | Self-care, Health. |
  BISAC: HEALTH & FITNESS / Healing. | SELF-HELP / Spiritual. | BODY,
MIND &
  SPIRIT / Healing / General.
Classification: LCC RC489.M53 B756 2018 (print) | LCC RC489.M53 (e-book) |
  DDC 616.89/1—dc23
LC record available at https://lccn.loc.gov/2018017232

Printed and bound in the Unites States

10 9 8 7 6 5 4 3 2

Edited by Jacqui Lewis
Text design and layout by Geoff Green Book Design CB24 4GL
This book was typeset in Kingfisher
Artwork by Jorgen Hojland

To send correspondence to the author of this book, mail a first-class letter to Annick Brofman c/o Inner Traditions • Bear & Company, One Park Street, Rochester, VT 05767, USA and we will forward the communication, or contact the Brofman Foundation directly at **https://brofman-foundation.org** or **angel@healer.ch**

A Note From Annick Brofman

Martin left this world on 11 August 2014, early morning, during a magnificent full moon. He devoted the last years of his life to the writing of this book, the third part of the work that he wanted to leave to the world before his departure.

Martin was an exceptional being, an extraordinary father to our son, and an extraordinary husband and mentor. The teachers he trained, of whom I am one, continue his work with pride. We admired the quality of his love and the clarity of his spirit, a model for ever.

I wrote down the story of Martin's departure, a synchronicity that illustrates the philosophies that are in this book and that we teach. You will find it on our website: https://brofman-foundation.org

We continue the path together, his soul at our side.

With love
Annick Brofman

My thanks to those students and others who asked about
so many of the symptoms listed, and who provided
positive feedback about the accuracy of the
analyses given them.

Thanks also to Dr Pierre Aubert (France) for reviewing the
list of medical descriptions for 'anomalies' –
and finding none.

Much appreciation for the constant encouragement and
support of the instructors of my methods, and of my
loving family, my wife Annick and my son Edouard.

Contents

Foreword

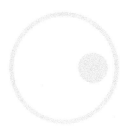

I knew Martin Brofman from 1980, when he came to give his first lecture in Europe, in Geneva. I had the privilege to be his first translator. And I was in total agreement with everything that he was saying. Being a holistic MD, I was happy to hear someone explaining that all our diseases start in our consciousness and that we cannot heal without working on it!

Over the years I was delighted to see how Martin, through his lectures and seminars in many countries, was able to give to many people these wonderful tools that have allowed them to become healers, for themselves and for others. And his teaching about the Body Mirror System of Healing has helped tens of thousands of practitioners to improve their ways of helping themselves and others.

I can enthusiastically recommend his book *Anything Can Be Healed* to anyone concerned with health and healing.

For half of his life, Martin was focused on quantifying the body/mind interface, and this book is the result of his inner and outer research during all this time, a vision of how symptoms and diseases are related to what is happening in the consciousness of the person affected.

As a medical doctor, I can vouch for the accuracy of the descriptions of the medical conditions. As someone also representing the alternative and complementary communities, I do enjoy the clarity of the explanations to the reader, no matter what their level of spiritual evolution – after all, it was written with the patient in mind who has the symptom, however useful it may also be for the helping professional.

I do believe that this book will be appreciated, not only by those who have already been in touch with Martin Brofman's teachings, but also by all those who are looking for a way to help themselves and others to go beyond a limited materialistic way of thinking in order to understand the value of what is happening in their life, at all levels. To grow in consciousness and happiness is the deep meaning of our lives on Planet Earth and this book will play an important role for all those who are concerned with spiritual progress, all those who want to walk into the light. We have been for some millennia living with fear, conflicts and diseases. It is time to step out of these nightmares, become awakened, taking responsibility for our lives in order to participate in the coming birth of a conscious humanity!

Dr. Christian Tal Schaller

Christian Tal Schaller, MD, has been working in pioneering European holistic medicine for more than forty years. Author of sixty books, he works with many health centres around the world and teaches in various countries, with his wife Johanne Razanamahay, that 'Health can be learned!' [www.santeglobale.info]

Preface

I am a cancer survivor. In 1975 was diagnosed with a spinal cord tumour that doctors had decided was inoperable and untreatable, and terminal. My right arm was paralyzed, my legs were spastic and I had sensations like electric shocks running along my spine and out to my extremities. I was given one or two months to live, unless I coughed or sneezed, in which case I could die in that moment. One year later, the same doctors decided they must have made a mistake, because there was no longer any evidence of the tumour nor its symptoms.

During the time between the original diagnosis and the revised version, I had been working on myself, doing inner work and exploring my consciousness, diligently applying myself as a full-time job, a matter of life and death. I used affirmations and visualizations, working at alpha levels of consciousness. I researched various Eastern philosophies and esoteric teachings, and came to understand more and more about the body/mind interface. With what I learned during the process of healing myself, I put together a model in my consciousness into which I could fit the various teachings I explored. This model came to be known as the Body Mirror System of Healing.

My first book about healing, *Anything Can Be Healed*, focuses on the dynamics of the Body Mirror System, and what is needed in order to function as a healer, and it also covers the basics of exploring the body as a map of the consciousness within. It eventually became apparent to me that there was a need for another book, focusing on what considerations are necessary in the consciousness of the healee, the person experiencing the symptoms and interested in healing himself or herself. This is the purpose of the book you are now reading. It documents the research I have been doing for the past thirty-eight years, quantifying the specific personality profiles associated with the various physical symptoms. While it is primarily intended for the person experiencing the symptom, it is at the same time very interesting for those in the helping professions, healers and therapists, to help them understand more fully the dynamics of the body/mind interface.

Since healing myself of the cancer in 1976, and continuing to dance with the variety of conditions presented to me by life, I have at times had to deal with and resolve various other symptoms that showed me that I had still more homework to do in order to remain in balance on all levels.

I have had a chance to look at my attitudes during my more recent experiences as well as during my first healing process, and make sense of what worked and what did not, and thus to further quantify the process of self-healing and the attitudes that could optimize the process. This book includes the result of this inner research, and also my observations and healing experiences with the tens of thousands of people I have worked with since 1976, in individual healings and in classes I have taught.

In fact, many of the symptoms included in this book were brought to my attention by the online discussion groups available to graduates of our classes, as well as by those people seeking advice in the free Healer's Message Board that has been available for years to those who have not attended our classes.

For the medical definitions and descriptions of the symptoms, various online medical dictionaries were also used for reference.

The personality profiles associated with the various symptoms are those derived from my own understanding of the chakras and the body/mind interface within the context of the Body Mirror System of Healing, and according to its concepts.

This book is intended as a reference to help readers understand the inner causes, the tensions in the consciousness that are associated with the various symptoms. The release of the tensions and how to accomplish this release is in the hands of the person experiencing the symptoms. Of course, knowing the relationship between the symptom and the corresponding inner cause can provide valuable insight into the options available to the person experiencing the symptom.

May you, the reader, find this book a valuable resource to help and understand those around you, and/or to facilitate your own healing, no matter what method you choose for that.

Anything can be healed.

Martin Brofman

Orientation

The Starting Point

Acceptance

Okay. You've got some kind of symptom. Whether you consider it to be the result of an accident, some organism, or just bad luck, you've got something to deal with, something to understand, some action to take.

Now what?

The diagnosis of a symptom, particularly one that may be considered life-threatening, can be a shock, with many strong emotions coming up for the person involved. Before any decisions are made in terms of how to proceed, the first step should be an emotional acceptance that the symptom exists.

Acceptance is not defeatism. It is not to say that by accepting the fact that the symptom exists, you are accepting that it will continue to its apparent logical conclusion. Emotionally accepting that the symptom exists simply gives you a starting point, from which you can decide what you want to do about it. You thus begin in a clear space. The symptom exists. It has been diagnosed on the physical level, as the result of some kind of physical or medical examination. That's a fact.

If someone has been diagnosed with a condition described as terminal, they have been given a medical opinion based on the result of a medical physical examination. It is important to emotionally accept the medical diagnosis, which is about the condition of the physical body at the moment it was examined, from the point of view of the medical establishment. It is also important to understand that the prognosis, the prediction according to the medical point of view about where the symptom may be heading, is an opinion based on the diagnosis. Any doctor will agree that getting another opinion is not only reasonable, but recommended. You can then see if there are differing opinions, or an agreed-upon diagnosis and prognosis for your condition.

If there is an agreed-upon prognosis by the medical establishment, if a number of doctors agree that this is the prognosis, the perceived eventual conclusion of the symptom, the person involved needs to get to grips with it and to accept emotionally that what the doctors have predicted is a distinct possibility. It might happen, and from the doctors' point of view, is very likely to happen. That needs to be emotionally accepted as a possibility. Once that is accepted emotionally, other possibilities can also be explored.

In my own case, I had to accept emotionally that the doctors expected me to die very soon from the spinal cord tumour I had experienced. When I did that, when I accepted the possibility of imminent death, releasing the fear of death, I was then more able to experience life more fully in the moment of experience. I was then able later to consider other possible futures, including the possibility of healing myself, and manifest that into reality.

An axiom among people working with their consciousness is that when you put certain pictures into your consciousness, you improve the probability of them happening. If you have a fear of something, then you continually put into your consciousness a picture of that thing happening. You are saying, 'I do not want that to happen.' The picture is clear. The fear of that happening is like glue attaching you to that picture.

If you have fear about the prognosis, you hold that picture in your consciousness about what might happen, and according to the dynamics of consciousness, you increase the possibility of that happening. If you are afraid to hear the doctor's opinion about what might in fact happen, you need to do something to release the fear, and thus dissolve the glue.

When you have emotionally accepted the possibility that what you have been afraid of might actually happen, you do dissolve the glue by releasing the fear, and you are then more easily able to hold your attention on what you want to happen, holding that picture in your consciousness, rather than what you have been afraid of happening. You get to grips with the symptom, and the diagnosis.

What happens next is up to you, your decision.

You can decide to follow the traditional medical approach and work with medical advice and treatment. I did that, and agreed to have an operation intended to remove the tumour, though afterwards I was told that it was not successful, and that the tumour was not accessible. That was when I was told that I had one or two months to live, unless I coughed or sneezed. I had to emotionally accept that as well, in order to eventually consider other possibilities.

You can decide to work with alternative or complementary approaches, and also with your consciousness, as I did. The methods you choose do not have to be considered mutually exclusive. You can use whatever makes sense to you, whatever it is you feel good using, in order to do something about the symptom.

It is important to understand that the symptom is not the problem – it is a symptom of the problem, an indication of the existence of something else. The medical view is that it is a sign or an indication of a disorder or a disease, and it can also be seen as an indication of the tensions in the consciousness that provides the environment in which the disorder or disease can exist, and which can then be seen as the inner cause.

This is explained more fully in the next chapter.

CHAPTER 2

The Inner Cause

Why did this symptom happen?

In terms of what you have decided to do about the symptom, whether you have made a decision to follow the traditional medical model, or use herbs, or energy work, or diet, or any other approach based on treating the symptom, it can be interesting to also consider why and how the symptom happened to you.

When we discuss the causes of physical symptoms, many people tend to think in terms of the physical cause, or what is seen as the cause in physical cause-and-effect reality. Of course symptoms manifest in physical reality, through accidents, injuries, microorganisms, etc. It is important, though, to also understand that the symptom would not have manifested if the conditions for it were not there in the person's consciousness.

For example, Type 'A' Behaviour is a personality profile that has been associated with heart disease. This means that there is a statistically significant correlation between people with Type 'A' Behaviour and those who develop heart disease. In other words, people with Type 'A' Behaviour have been seen to be more likely than others to develop heart disease. We can say that Type 'A' Behaviour is a heart disease personality. Whatever might be seen as the physical cause of heart disease, it is acknowledged that this personality type is a consistent element.

There is also a cancer personality, a near-sighted personality, an arthritis personality, etc. In fact, every physical symptom can be associated with a particular way of being. If you have a symptom, you have a way of being that correlates with that symptom.

The way of being associated with the symptom is not who you are, but rather a way of being you have adopted as the result of decisions you have made in response to events in your life. If you were not born with the symptom, you were not born with that way of being. Rather, it reflects decisions you made in your life in response to conditions at that time, and the stressed way of being with which you have identified since then.

If it was a symptom evident at birth, it was still reflecting tension in your consciousness about conditions in your life at that time; the decisions made at that time, at no matter which level, can still be changed, and those tensions released, to return to a way of being that more truly reflects who you really are.

The symptom on the physical level reflects tension in your consciousness about something that was happening in your life at the time the symptom began.

You made decisions in response to conditions in your life at that time, decisions that left you with stress, and which encouraged a way of being that correlates with the symptom that developed. In that way, it can be said that the way of being you adopted attracted or nourished that symptom, regardless of the apparent cause on the physical level.

If you have a stressed way of being that has resulted in a physical symptom, it is important to emphasize again that the way of being you have been experiencing is not who you really are, but just what you have been doing, a reflection of the way you have chosen to respond to conditions around you. You can make different choices. There is always a choice.

No matter which methods you have decided to use to treat or release the symptom, you can also decide to release the stressed way of being associated with the symptom, which can be seen as the inner cause of the symptom. If the decisions you have made have resulted in a stressed way of being, if you have created a personality profile associated with a particular symptom, then it follows that it is possible to release the stressed way of being, the personality profile that attracted the symptom. You can change your mind about something, and interact with your environment in a different way that is not as stressed, and that more reflects who you really are.

The effect of doing that can be to encourage the release of the symptom, since the environment that attracted or nourished it no longer exists to sustain it. By releasing the stress, and the stressed way of being, the inner cause, you can be more assured that the symptom will not have a tendency to return.

In this way, the process of healing implies a process of transformation, a release of a way of being that is not who you really are, and a return to who you really are, the real you.

We can explore the mechanism behind this process.

Everything begins with your consciousness

Let's look at what this means.

You are inside there, inside your body, looking out through your eyes, and things happen around you. It is you who decides what to think, what to feel and how to respond to these conditions.

The 'you' who is doing this deciding is what we are calling your consciousness.

The way you choose to respond – and there is always a choice – can leave you in balance, or can leave you with stress. When it leaves you with stress, you are out of balance in your consciousness. There is tension in your consciousness about something happening in your life at that time.

If the tension reaches a certain level of intensity, it can result in a symptom on the physical level. The symptom speaks a language, and this language reflects the idea that we create our reality, and points to what we consider to be the inner cause of the symptom.

We will be exploring this idea further. For now, we can say that on some level, the symptom served a positive purpose in terms of helping you to understand yourself and your response to life. The symptom was a message from a deeper part of your consciousness about tension you were holding about a situation in your life that needed to be resolved at that time.

We create our reality

Symptoms are the result of stress. When we are exploring the inner cause of the symptom, we consider that we have created the symptom through the stressed way we chose to respond to the conditions in our life at the time the symptom developed or was discovered.

When we say that we have created the symptom, it doesn't mean that we have consciously chosen to have that symptom, but rather that the symptom was the logical conclusion of the particular thoughts and emotions we chose that left us with stress, and that resulted in the symptom.

It's not something to feel guilty about, but rather to understand as a logical process, in order to choose to make different decisions, choosing different thoughts and emotions, different perceptions that could have the effect of releasing the inner cause, the stressed way of thinking that created the symptom. If the symptom served to give us a message, once we have got the message and changed something accordingly, then the symptom has no further reason for being there and can be released, according to whatever we can allow ourselves to believe is possible.

The symptom speaks a language that reflects the idea that we create our reality. Whether or not we really understand the full meaning of that statement, that we create our reality, it is interesting to use the model as a way to understand what the symptom has been telling us about the stressed way we have chosen to respond to the conditions in our life at the time the symptom began. The metaphor of the symptom becomes evident. We can see how it can make sense to us, how we can recognize ourselves in the metaphor.

When I had the tumour I could have said that I was paralyzed, and that I had difficulty walking. Changing the words in order to describe the symptom from the point of view that I created it, I would have said that I had been keeping myself from walking – in other words, I had been keeping myself from leaving a situation in which I had been unhappy. The deep part of me had wanted to walk away, but I had been giving myself reasons to stay in that unhappy situation, and the stress of doing that had reached catastrophic proportions in my body.

I recognized myself in that explanation.

Rather than saying that I was paralyzed, I would have to say that I had been paralyzing myself. In other words, I had been trying to be what I thought others wanted me to be, holding back the real me, and, again, the stress of that had reached catastrophic proportions in my body. Again, I recognized myself in the explanation, and therefore I knew that I needed to do something different. My body was saying, 'This is what you have been doing to yourself.'

If you have a symptom, that symptom on the physical level began with and reflected a certain tension in your consciousness about what was happening in your life at the time the symptom began or was detected.

By seeing things from this point of view, you can take responsibility for the symptom.

This is about responsibility without guilt. It's not about beating yourself up about having created the symptom – it's about understanding that if you decided to think in a certain way which then created the symptom, then deciding to think differently can be part of releasing the symptom. It's strictly mechanics – cause and effect.

It is an empowering point of view.

When you take responsibility for the symptom, you put yourself in the driver's seat. You are no longer the victim, with things happening to you that you can do nothing about. You can do something about it by changing your mind about something, by choosing another way of thinking or acting, which can have the effect of releasing the stress in your consciousness that had been associated with the symptom.

That's what I did, and what worked for me.

'Terminal' conditions

Working with the idea that everything begins in your consciousness, if you have developed a symptom that could have death as its logical conclusion, it follows that the symptom must have begun with a deep decision to die. Typically, anyone with a symptom diagnosed as terminal has been facing a situation in their life that they find unacceptable but see no way out of, except to die. If we understand that, it follows that the body has been carrying out the individual's wishes, and the kind of symptom can tell a story about the reasons for not wanting to go on.

It also follows that if the individual can make a different deep decision, based on finding a way out of or resolving the situation they had seen as unacceptable, and releasing the tensions from their consciousness, their body will then be able to carry out the new decision by releasing the symptom that had been based on the old perceptions and their associated tensions.

We can say that the symptom on the physical level has been a reflection of the deeper part of your consciousness, the part that we refer to as the spirit, which the Western traditions know as the 'unconscious' or 'subconscious'. When you do not find a way to resolve something in your everyday consciousness, something about which you feel tension, you put it away in this deeper part of your consciousness, your spirit, where it is still running in the background. It is this tension running in the background that creates the symptom on the physical level.

It is this deeper part of your consciousness, your spirit, that is the real you, your higher self, the part of your consciousness that has been directing your life. It is this deep part of you that has been telling you through the symptom, 'This is what you have been doing to yourself.'

The implication is that you can do something different.

You can decide to do something that can have the effect of releasing the symptom.

Then, you can decide what to do.

The Body/Mind Interface

The Human Directional System

You are guided from within, by means of what you may know as your intuition, or your instinct. It speaks a simple language. Either it feels good, or it doesn't. Everything else is politics.

We are told that if you listen to this inner voice, this inner sense of knowing, it leads you to success and fulfilment. Do what feels right, and you are doing the right thing. If it doesn't feel right, we are told, you should not do it.

You can listen to this inner sense of direction by instinctively doing what feels right – or you can do it through an inner dialogue. You can ask inside, 'How does it feel if I move in this direction?' 'How does it feel if I go in that direction?' One direction may feel more flowing, while the other might feel as though there is more resistance. See which feels better to you, and trust it.

If for some reason you decide to move in the direction of resistance ('Well, I need to be sure' or 'People would want me to do this instead'), the inner voice has to get louder.

The next level of communication is the emotions. As you move more in the direction of resistance, you feel more and more resistance. You feel more and more emotions that do not feel good, and you can also see the resistance in terms of things that have a tendency not to happen. There is resistance to them happening.

At some point, you can say, 'Stop. Look. Listen. I should have listened to my feelings, to the little voice inside that said to do the other thing.' That means you heard the little voice. Otherwise, you would not have been able to say, 'I should have listened.'

At this point you can change your mind and move in the direction of the flow, in the direction of what feels better. Then there is more of a feeling of aliveness; things have a tendency to feel better, and to flow more easily, and you know you are on the right path again.

If for some reason you continue to move in the direction of the resistance ('Well, I promised' or 'Conditions are not yet right to make the change,' etc.), the inner communication gets louder, and the next level is the physical body. You create a symptom. The symptom speaks a language that reflects the idea that you create your reality. When you describe it from that point of view, the metaphor of the symptom becomes clear. The symptom is the mechanism for the communication from the deep part of who you are, about what you have been doing to yourself, that is different from what that part of you, the real you, your spirit, really wants to do.

Thus, the levels of communication from your Higher Self to the level of your personality in the body/mind interface are:

1. Intuition > 2. Emotion > 3. Physical Body

The symptom on the physical level must manifest through physical reality, through some 'accident', for example, or some microorganism. The means of manifestation are not as important as the end result, the symptom itself, and what it has been communicating. If the symptom is the result of an accident, for example, we can ask what guided you to be in that situation. If the symptom was the result of what you ate, we can ask what guided you to eat that. If the symptom was the result of some microorganism, we can ask why you were affected by it, when some others were not – or what guided you to be in that place at that time to attract that organism. Remember that you are always guided by your spirit.

The symptom served to tell you something about unresolved tension in your consciousness about something that was happening in your life at that time.

Specific symptoms on the physical level reflect specific tensions in your consciousness, and specific ways of being that are related to the symptoms.

When you do something that is different from what the symptom says you have been doing, then you have got the message of the symptom on some level and understood it. The symptom then has no further reason for being there, and it can be released, according to whatever you allow yourself to believe is possible.

You Are An Energy System

Your consciousness, your experience of being, who you really are, is energy. You might think of it as 'life energy.' This energy, your consciousness, does not just live in your brain. It fills your entire body. Your consciousness is connected to every cell in your body. Through your consciousness, you can communicate with every organ and every tissue, and a number of therapies are based on this communication with whichever organs have been affected by some kind of symptom or disorder.

This energy, which is your consciousness and which reflects your state of being, can be measured through the process known as Kirlian photography. When you take a Kirlian photograph of your hand, it shows a certain pattern of energy. If you take a second photograph while imagining that you are sending love and energy to someone you know, the Kirlian photograph will show a different pattern of energy. Thus, we can see that a change in your consciousness creates a change in the energy field that is being photographed, which we call the aura.

This energy field has been quantified so that 'holes' in particular parts of the energy field correspond to particular weaknesses in specific parts of the physical body. The interesting thing about this is that the weakness consistently shows up in the energy field before there is any evidence of it on the physical level.

The direction of manifestation is very interesting.

1. A change of consciousness creates a change in the energy field.

2. A change in the energy field happens before a change in the physical body.

The direction of manifestation is from the consciousness, through the energy field, to the physical body.

1. Consciousness ❯ 2. Energy Field ❯ 3. Physical Body

When we look at things in this way, we see that it is not the physical body creating the energy field, the aura, but rather the aura or energy field that is creating the physical body. What we see as the physical body is the end result of a process that begins with the consciousness.

When you make a decision that leaves you with stress, it affects your consciousness, and therefore your energy field. When the tension increases to a certain degree of intensity, it reaches the physical level, and you create a symptom.

That means that if you make a different decision, change your mind about something or resolve a situation that you have previously responded to with stress, releasing the inner tension, that change can affect your energy field in a different way, and the symptom can be released, in accord with your beliefs about what is possible.

Even when the release of the symptom is accomplished through classical medical technology, we can still say that making the inner changes described above can give more of an assurance that the symptom will not be recreated, and that the part of the body or function within the body that had been affected is less likely to be affected again in the future.

Anyway, you will be happier, having released tensions from your consciousness and taking charge of your life.

Of course, if you are working with alternative or complementary methods, you have considered that the release of the symptom can happen – or be accelerated – through these other means, be they physical or metaphysical, using herbs or diet, energy work or self-development tools.

Work with whatever makes sense to you, whatever resonates with you, whatever talks to you.

All the methods work for someone – and they can work for you, as well.

Reading the Body as a Map of the Consciousness

Tensions in the physical body reflect tensions in the consciousness about something happening in the person's life at the time the symptom began, and this process is quantifiable. Specific symptoms are related to specific tensions in the consciousness, which we can see as the inner cause of the symptom.

If someone wants to release a symptom, they can release the way of being that is associated with the symptom, the inner cause. To understand the inner cause of physical symptoms, the body can be seen as representing a map of the consciousness within. Tensions in a particular part of the physical body reflect specific tensions in the consciousness. An understanding of the energy centres known as 'chakras' gives us the key to reading this map.

The chakras regulate the flow of energy through the energy system of which we are each composed.

We are each an energy field, an energy system, energy in a state of movement.

In the balanced and healthy individual, the energy flows freely. When we make a decision that leaves us with tension, we block the flow of energy. It no longer flows freely.

When the tension reaches a certain degree of intensity, we can create a symptom on the physical level.

Thus, we can say that all physical symptoms can be seen as blocked energy. All illness, all injury, can be seen and understood as just blocked energy.

Restoring the flow of energy and returning to our natural state of balance and wholeness can be accomplished by changing our mind about something, making a different decision, releasing the inner tension, the inner cause, and seeing the effects of that on the physical level as a release of the symptom.

The Chakras

Chakra is a Sanskrit word meaning wheel, or vortex, and it refers to each of the seven energy centres of which our consciousness, our energy system, is composed. These chakras, or energy centres, function as pumps or valves, regulating the flow of energy through our energy system. The functioning of the chakras reflects decisions we make concerning how we choose to perceive and respond to conditions in our life. We open and close these valves when we decide what to think, and what to feel, and through which perceptual filter we choose to experience events in the world around us.

The chakras are not physical, but that doesn't mean that they are not real. They are aspects of consciousness in the same way that the auras are aspects of consciousness. The chakras are more dense than the auras, but not as dense as the physical body. The chakras interact with the physical body through two major vehicles, the endocrine system and the nervous system.

Each of the seven chakras is associated with one of the seven endocrine glands, and these control the chemical balance in your body. Each chakra is also associated with a group of nerves called a plexus. Each plexus controls certain parts of the body and certain functions within the body. Thus, each chakra can be associated with particular parts of the body and particular functions within the body controlled by that plexus, and with the endocrine gland associated with that chakra.

All of your senses, all of your perceptions, all of your possible states of awareness, everything that is possible for you to experience, can be divided into seven categories. Each category, each portion of your consciousness, can be associated with a particular chakra. Thus, the chakras represent not only particular parts of your physical body, but also particular parts of your consciousness.

When you feel tension in your consciousness about something happening around you, you feel it in a particular part of your body depending on the reason for the tension. Where you feel the tension depends upon why you feel the tension. You feel it in the chakra associated with that part of your consciousness experiencing the stress, and in the parts of the physical body associated with that chakra.

The tension in the chakra is detected by the nerves of the plexus associated with that chakra, and then transmitted to the parts of the body controlled by that plexus, that group of nerves. Thus, tensions in the consciousness are experienced as tensions in the physical body.

So, if you are faced with a perceived threat to your survival, the fear located in one of the chakras (the root chakra) stimulates the adrenal glands, preparing you for fight or flight; and because the parts of the body associated with that chakra include the legs, your legs may shake in fear.

When the tension continues over a period of time, or to a particular level of intensity, it may create a symptom on the physical level. With the example just given, the symptom might be problems with the legs.

Following this model, we can say that when you have a symptom on the physical level, that physical symptom reflects tension in your consciousness about something happening in your life at that time, and the tension about what is happening is experienced in the chakra associated with that specific part of your consciousness, and that part of your physical body associated with that chakra and thus experiencing the symptom.

What we show briefly in the summary below represents the relationship between the various parts of the body and the corresponding parts of the consciousness for each chakra. A much more detailed and complete analysis can be found in later sections of this book. Other more esoteric aspects of the consciousness (such as associations with various subtle bodies, colours, musical notes) are not included because they do not directly relate to the body/mind interface – though they are mentioned in the Chakra Reference Chart at the end of the book.

If you have been experiencing a symptom, you will see that this summary points you to the tension in your consciousness that you can associate with the symptom on the physical level, in terms of what was happening in your life at the time the symptom began. You know what you have been feeling good about and what you have been feeling tension about. You are the expert in what has been happening in your own consciousness.

Red Chakra (Root Chakra)

> **Parts of the body** – Legs, elimination system, skeletal system, lymph system, adrenal glands. Sense of smell. Nose. Teeth and gums.
>
> **Parts of the consciousness** – Security, survival, trust; the parts of your life having to do with safety.

Tensions in this chakra can be experienced as fear, insecurity or mistrust, and can be related to tensions about the home, about money or work, difficulty letting in love from one's mother. Often, a person's relationship with their mother sets the pattern for their relationship with everything that represents security.

Orange Chakra (Sacral Chakra)

Parts of the body – Gonads, sense of taste. Sexual organs and glands. Tongue.

Parts of the consciousness – Relationship with food, sex and having children.

Tensions in this chakra can be related to tension or ambivalence about sex or having children, or the person not listening to what their body is asking for in terms of food or sex.

Yellow Chakra (Solar Plexus Chakra)

Parts of the body – All organs located mid-body, as well as skin, muscles, jaw. Eyes. Sense of sight.

Parts of the consciousness – Power, control, freedom. Ease of being.

Tension in the solar plexus can be related to anger or control issues, or tension about freedom, or how the person feels about how they are seen by others.

Green Chakra (Heart Chakra)

Parts of the body – Heart, blood circulatory system, lungs, thymus gland, immune system. Sense of touch.

Parts of the consciousness – Perceptions of love, the area of relationships, people close to your heart, like partners, parents, siblings, children.

Tensions in this chakra reflect conflict or disappointment with someone close, not feeling loved or tensions about being in a relationship (or not being in one).

Blue Chakra (Throat Chakra)

Parts of the body – Throat, arms, wrists, hands, fingers, thyroid gland, ears, sense of hearing.

Parts of the consciousness – Expressing, receiving, communicating, setting goals.

Tensions in this chakra could be experienced as difficulty communicating or expressing oneself, or difficulty expressing emotions.

Indigo Chakra (Brow Chakra)

Parts of the body – Forehead, pituitary gland, trigeminal nerves, carotid plexus.

Parts of the consciousness – Spirit (unconscious, subconscious), subtle senses (ESP like clairvoyance, clairaudience, etc.).

Tensions in this chakra could be experienced as not listening to one's inner voice, or not feeling at ease with one's body, or having felt a deep conflict about not being seen for who one is.

Violet Chakra (Crown Chakra)

Parts of the body – Brain, head, hair, nervous system, pineal gland.

Parts of the consciousness – Unity versus isolation, sense of direction, connection with father, authority.

Tensions in this chakra could be experienced as conflict with authority and/or feeling isolated or separated from someone close. Often, the person's relationship with their father establishes the pattern for their relationship with authority and with their god(s).

Yin and Yang

In reading the body as a map of the consciousness within, it is important to pay attention to which side of the body is affected. We have a right side and a left side, which can be described as a yang side and a yin side, or male and female sides (yang = male, yin = female), or acting and feeling sides (yang = acting, yin = feeling), or also will and emotional sides (yang = will, yin = emotions).

Yang	Yin
Male	Female
Acting	Feeling
Will	Emotions

For people born right-handed, their right side is their yang side. For those born left-handed, their left side is their yang side, even if they have learned to use their right side as their dominant side.

Thus, most people's right leg would be their male, will and acting leg, and their left leg would be their female, emotional, feeling leg. For those born left-handed, the polarity would be reversed, and their left leg would be their male, will or acting leg, and their right leg would be their female, emotional, feeling leg.

The Effect of the Symptom

It is important to consider not only the symptom itself, but also how the person feels affected by it; then the words they use can be rearranged or altered to reflect the idea that the person created it.

Thus, instead of the person saying, 'I can't walk,' it could be said that the person has been metaphorically keeping themselves from walking – keeping themselves from leaving a situation in which they feel unhappy. Instead of saying, 'I can't see,' it could be said that they have been keeping themselves from seeing something, or avoiding looking at something – within the context of what was happening in their life at the time the symptom began. The symptom can be seen as a metaphor for what the person has been doing to him/herself – a message from the deep part of their consciousness that is known as the spirit, or the higher self, or in the Western traditions as the unconscious or subconscious.

When we see this principle in action, it is more and more evident to what degree we really do create our reality.

Questions to Ask

Now that you have a sense of how things work, and have emotionally accepted that the symptom exists and are willing to see what it is in your consciousness that attracted or nurtured the symptom, the next step is to ask yourself some questions.

What do the symptoms say about the tension in your consciousness?

What was happening in your life at the time the symptom began?

When you see that you were stressed about events in your life at the time the symptom appeared or was diagnosed, you can see the relationship between the stress in your consciousness and the symptom on the physical level.

Sometimes the symptom is discovered at a certain time, but you are told that it must have been there for years, or perhaps even that you were born with it. In such cases, it is still significant to work with the time it was discovered or diagnosed, and to look at what was happening in your life at that time.

If you have been told that it started some time before the diagnosis or discovery, you can also look at what was happening in your life at that time, and see the parallels with what was happening later, when the symptom was discovered or diagnosed; this will probably make sense to you as well. Or you may be able to see that some sensitivity was established at that earlier time, which relates to and was touched or triggered by events at the later time of diagnosis.

It is not helpful to get involved with stories about symptoms coming from past lives, because that does not answer the question of why the symptom appeared at that specific time in your life. In the same way, stories of symptoms being inherited do not answer the question of why the symptom manifested at a certain age. We are interested in what was happening in your life at the time the symptom began; this will make evident a much more coherent explanation.

The message of the symptom gives you a sense of what parts of your life you can look at. For example, if your legs were affected, you can look at what was happening in the root chakra parts of your life at that time (money, home, work), since the legs are associated with the root chakra. If your heart was affected, you can look at tensions in the area of relationships at that time.

What is the message or metaphor of the symptom?

You can check out the message or metaphor of the symptom by searching through the reference section of this book according to the part(s) of the body affected, the function affected or the name of the symptom. That will give you a sense of the tension in the consciousness that is associated with the symptom – the personality profile that the symptom represents, and which we understand as the inner cause.

Generally speaking, when looking for the message of the symptom, first consider the part of the body that is affected, and see what function has been affected. How do you experience the symptom? What activities or functions (breathing, walking, seeing, etc.) are affected? Describe it from the point of view that you created it, and see how that makes sense as a metaphor for what you have been doing to yourself, how you had responded to events at the time the symptom began. For example, if your walking is affected, you can ask yourself what unhappy situation you have been keeping yourself from walking away from. If your vision has been affected, what have you had resistance to seeing or looking at? If it is your throat, what is it that you have been avoiding to express or communicate?

Which chakra(s) have been involved?

Which chakra is associated with the part of the body or function within the body that has been affected by the symptom?

Each chakra is associated with a particular part of your consciousness about a specific part of your life. Thus:

Root chakra — money, home, work

Sacral chakra — food, sex, having children

Solar plexus chakra — power, control, freedom

Heart chakra — relationships, people close to your heart

Throat chakra — expressing, communicating

Brow chakra — spirituality, non-ordinary perceptions

Crown chakra — tensions with father/authority, or a sense of separation from someone close

See which chakra(s) have been involved with the symptom, and you will be able to identify the tensions in the specific parts of your consciousness about the particular parts of your life that these chakras represent. See how you can relate to or remember having experienced these tensions in your consciousness at the time the symptom began, in response to what had been happening in your life at that time. If you do not remember the situation directly, you can still know or remember historically what was happening in your life at that time and ask yourself, looking at the situation from the outside, how you might imagine the character in the scene (you) reacting to that situation.

Once you recognize these tensions in your consciousness about the situation you were in at that time, it will be easier to recognize that they are related to your physical symptom. It could logically follow, then, that if the tensions in your consciousness had something to do with the symptoms in your body, releasing the tensions from your consciousness could make it easier to release the physical symptoms that had been their effect.

How have you felt affected by the symptom?

What do you feel the symptom has been preventing you from doing? What activities have been affected? Describe them to yourself. Then, describe them from the point of view that you have created the symptom. Rather than saying, 'I can't...', you can say, 'I have been keeping myself from...' and see how that makes sense to you.

For example, if you say, 'I can't walk,' you can ask yourself what unhappy situation you have been giving yourself reasons to stay in, thus keeping yourself from walking away. If the effect of the symptom has been that you feel helpless, ask yourself how you have been making yourself helpless in the way you have been talking to yourself, saying, 'I can't.' If you have had difficulty speaking, or if that could be the logical conclusion of the symptom if it were allowed to continue, you can ask yourself what it is that you had been keeping yourself from expressing or communicating.

Note that in looking at the effect of the symptom, it is important to look not only at how you have been affected until now, but how you would be affected if the symptom were allowed to proceed to its logical conclusion. If your shoulder hurts, for example, and that were allowed to go to its logical conclusion, the result would be an inability to move that arm, and it could then be said that you would be unable to reach for something. Described from the point of view that you created it, and looking at what could be the inner cause in your consciousness, it could then be said that you have been keeping yourself from reaching for something. In that case, there must have been something there, something to reach for, a goal that existed, some picture in the future, but the way you had been talking to yourself inside had discouraged you from going for it.

What can you do about the situation and/or the tensions?

When you can see a connection between the symptom and the events in your life at the time the symptom appeared or was discovered, you can better understand how the symptom can be viewed as the manifestation on the physical level of the stress or tension in your consciousness about what was happening in your life at that time. Then you will also see that it is important to release the tensions from your consciousness, and the possible beliefs you may have created with decisions you made at that time.

You have various options in terms of releasing the tensions in your consciousness:

A. If you recognize that you had created a belief ('Men are not to be trusted' or, 'I'll never find love', for example) you can make a different decision ('THAT man is not to be trusted' or 'Love is all around. I just need to recognize it', for example).
B. You can change the situation so that it is no longer stressful for you. For example, if your home doesn't feel safe, ask yourself what you can do to make it safe.

C. You can change the way you look at the situation. Reframe it. Seeing it in a new light can change your attitude toward it, and in that way the stress can be released. For example, if it looked at the time as though there was no love there, you can replay the situation, adding the missing ingredient. How would it look if you knew you were loved? It will then make sense in a different way.

D. Leave the situation, so that you are not in the middle of something every day that you are not happy with. Own your freedom and your power to decide for yourself what to do and how to live your life.

Specific possibilities are presented in the reference section of this book, related to specific symptoms. For example, cancer represents something held in and not expressed and the part of the body affected shows what this was – so the message would be to express what you had not been expressing. If it had been a question of holding back your sexuality, then express it. If you had been keeping yourself from communicating, then start communicating. If the symptom had been about not letting love in, decide to let the love in.

You can do the opposite of what the symptom says you had been doing, knowing that the symptom has been a message from your higher self, the real you, letting you know what you had been doing to yourself – so when you do something different, the symptom will have no further reason for being there, and it can be released according to whatever you allow yourself to believe is possible, either through inner work, or classical medicine, or whatever fits into your personal belief system.

If you have had a problem with your right eye, for example, and you are right-handed, we can say that it has something to do with your will eye, or your male eye. Thus, we can say that you have been keeping yourself from seeing what you want, or not seeing the male in your life, feeling separated from men or a man in your life, in terms of what was happening at the time the symptom began. That reflects a belief that you can change.

If you have had a problem with your elimination system, we would ask what was happening in the root chakra areas of your life – money, home, work – at the time the symptom began, and see what needs to be resolved there.

A problem with the skin over the heart area would say something about solar plexus energy (anger, for example) in the area of relationships, since the skin is related to the solar plexus chakra, and the heart is about the area of relationships, people close to your heart and your perceptions of love.

If there is a symptom that can be related to tensions with your mother, it makes sense to release the tensions for your own health and well-being, since with them you have only been hurting yourself.

The reference section of this book goes into much more detail concerning specific symptoms and the tensions in the consciousness that are associated with these symptoms. When you read the personality profile associated with a symptom you have been experiencing, the inner cause, you can just ask yourself if it talks to you, if you can recognize yourself in what is being described. When you recognize that the specific tensions being described are what you can relate to from what you experienced at the time the symptom began, that will show you the possibilities open to you of releasing those tensions, and thus releasing the effects of those tensions.

One way or another, just do whatever you can, in whatever way is comfortable for you, to release the symptom, heal it, cure it and return to your natural state of clarity, balance and health.

Get it healed

Heal yourself

Resolve the situation

Change your mind

Release the tension

An A–Z Guide to Symptoms and Conditions

Abcess – See Abscess

Abdomen

While the abdomen technically refers to the area between the thorax and the pelvis, this term is used here to refer to the lower abdomen – the area between the solar plexus and the pelvis. According to our map, the upper abdomen will be referred to as the solar plexus area.

The lower abdomen corresponds to the location of the sacral (second, orange) chakra, and is therefore related to the parts of the person's consciousness concerned with food, sex and having children.

Tensions on the will side (right side for right-handed people) would represent a conflict between the person's will and what their body is asking for in these areas, and tension on the emotional side would point to an emotional conflict about what the body is asking for.

If the symptom affects any part of the large or small intestine, there may be relevance to its relationship with food, and also with the person's elimination system (which is connected with the root chakra); tensions here may also be possibly related to sex or having children. For example, symptoms affecting the appendix in an adolescent can point to a conflict between their will and what their body is asking for in terms of food, but can also indicate insecurities – tensions in the root chakra – in the area of what the person's body is asking for in terms of sex.

Tensions about food, sex or having children can also manifest in the back at the level of the lumbar plexus, the 'small of the back'.

Because the sacral chakra is also associated with the emotional body, and the person's willingness to feel their emotions, symptoms may indicate that the person experienced a strong emotional shock at the time the symptom began. When this happens, the person may decide not to feel those emotions by shutting down their sacral chakra, thus turning off the other aspects of the chakra. This may affect them in terms of their appetite or their sexuality.

Abdominal cramps

Cramps or pain may occur when any of the muscles in the abdomen or in the walls of the bowels are stretched or strained. Because many internal organs are located in this region, it is important to know the location of the cramping relative to the closest chakra, or know what organs are involved, in order to determine the inner cause.

For example, if it is the stomach that is affected, that points to the solar plexus chakra and issues of power or control, while lower abdominal cramps during the menstrual cycle could point to tensions about not being pregnant, or about feeling that there is a disadvantage to being female.

Abortion

An abortion is the medical process of ending a pregnancy so it does not result in the birth of a baby. The term 'spontaneous abortion' refers to miscarriage, a naturally occurring event, and not to medical abortions or surgical abortions.

Whether or not the termination of pregnancy is the result of a medical procedure, it reflects the woman's desire to be a mother (or she would not have become pregnant), though not to have the child with the conditions in her life at the time of that pregnancy.

Abrasions – See Bruises/Abrasions

Abscess

An abscess is a collection of pus that has accumulated in a cavity formed by the tissue due to an infectious process (usually caused by bacteria or parasites) or other foreign materials (e.g. splinters, bullet wounds or injections from needles). It is a defensive reaction of the tissue to prevent the spread of infectious materials to other parts of the body.

The organisms or foreign materials kill the local cells, resulting in the release of toxins. The toxins trigger an inflammatory response, which draws large numbers of white blood cells to the area and increases the regional blood flow.

Because the abscess is an inflammation, or irritation, it implies anger, and the part of the body affected reflects what the irritation or anger is about.

Accident

According to the Human Directional System described in Chapter 3 of this book, there are no accidents and no coincidences. Things happen according to a pattern and an order that is related to what has been happening in the consciousness of the person involved in the event. The end result of the 'accident' was the real original intention. If the 'accident' resulted in a symptom, then the person was guided to that event in order to have that symptom, in order to show them which part of their consciousness was holding tension about a situation in their life that needed to be resolved. The symptom on the physical level reflects tension in the person's consciousness about something happening in their life at the time the symptom began or was discovered.

Achalasia

Achalasia, also known as oesophageal achalasia, achalasia cardiae, cardiospasm and oesophageal aperistalsis, is a disorder involving the smooth muscle layer of the oesophagus and the lower oesophageal sphincter. It is caused by the inability of smooth muscle to move food down the oesophagus. Achalasia is characterized by difficulty swallowing, regurgitation and sometimes chest pain.

Because the tensions involve the chest and stomach, the symptom is associated with tensions in the heart chakra and solar plexus chakra, pointing to issues of control in the area of relationships. The person finds a certain situation with someone close to their heart 'hard to swallow'. These tensions could also be related to Acid Reflux (below).

Acid Indigestion – See Heartburn

Acid Reflux

Acid reflux is a condition in which stomach acids rise up into the oesophagus because the valve that separates the stomach contents from the oesophagus is faulty. This can be due to the lower oesophageal sphincter not working properly, or a hiatus hernia.

This symptom represents the person having difficulty moving their attention between their solar plexus chakra and their heart chakra, because of tensions held in the solar plexus chakra. The person would like to hold their attention on perceptions of love but is having difficulty because of issues of power, control, freedom and possibly anger affecting the area of relationships.

Acidosis

Acidosis is characterized by high levels of acid waste products in the blood. Metabolic acidosis usually causes rapid breathing. Confusion or lethargy may also occur.

Breathing difficulties point to tensions in the area of the heart chakra and therefore relationships, and the lethargy can point to tensions in the areas associated with the root chakra – money, home, work. Therefore, this combination of symptoms can point to tensions with someone close to the person's heart, at home.

Because there are many types of acidosis, and many ways in which the person can experience the effects, see the particular symptoms experienced by the person, and the parts of the body affected, in order to see more precisely which tensions in the consciousness are associated with those particular symptoms.

Acne Vulgaris

Acne generally affects the skin on the face, and is considered unattractive. From the point of view that we each create our reality, the person affected has been making themselves unattractive. The symptom is designed to keep others, particularly potential partners, at a distance. As a skin problem, the symptom points to the solar plexus chakra, but has its effect in other areas, including the area of relationships and/or sexuality. The person is keeping potential partners at a distance because of sensitivities in the area of freedom or being themselves in relationships or sexual activities.

If the acne is on other parts of the body not generally visible when the person is wearing clothes, the sensitivities can relate to intimate contact. The person could be sensitive about removing their clothes. It is not the acne creating the sensitivities; rather it is the sensitivities creating the acne.

Acne on the shoulders could also point to unexpressed anger manifesting as an irritation.

Acromegaly (Gigantism)

Gigantism is abnormal growth due to an excess of growth hormone during childhood; it points to tensions in the brow chakra, and possibly the person not being happy to be in their body. The additional possible symptoms of headaches (crown chakra tensions) and increased sweating (elimination system – root chakra) raise questions of what was happening in the person's family life at home at the time the symptom began, in relation to tensions with their parents, and possibly feeling particularly conspicuous and isolated, since that is one of the effects of the symptom.

When it occurs in adulthood it is usually caused by a tumour in the pituitary gland, and may be accompanied by headaches. This points to tensions in a deep part of the person's consciousness (brow chakra), and feelings of isolation and separation (crown chakra) in response to conditions in the person's life at the time the symptom began. Bone growth in the face and body can also reflect root chakra tensions concerning home, and solar plexus chakra issues concerning the person's insecurity about their image, and having felt conspicuous and/or unattractive at the time in their life when the symptom first began.

Acute Myocardial Infarction (AMI)

Myocardial infarction (MI) or acute myocardial infarction (AMI), commonly known as a heart attack, results from the interruption of blood supply to a part of the heart, causing heart cells to die. It is related to the heart chakra, and therefore the area of relationships, reflecting tensions or a shock concerning someone close to the person's heart (a partner, parent, sibling or child) with the decision being made that the resulting tension is unacceptable and that the person doesn't want to face life with that situation as it is.

Addiction

Addictions or dependencies can point to tensions in various chakras, depending on the nature of the addiction. Although one usually considers addiction to be linked to substance abuse, the difficulty is not with the substance itself, but rather the addictive personality, and the chakra involved with the dependency gives a clearer idea of the true nature of the addiction.

A keen enjoyment of something does not equate to an addiction, though some might see it as one. An addiction is measured by the difficult emotions a person feels when they do not get what they want. The intensity of the difficult emotions shows the degree of the dependency. If the person does not feel bad when they do not get the substance, they are not addicted.

The anticipated effect of the 'substance abuse' gives a clue to the chakra involved. For example, if the liver is affected by alcohol abuse, it is related to the solar plexus chakra, and issues of power, control or freedom. Tension in the solar plexus is often experienced as anger or holding on to control. The person is unhappy about something happening in their life, and feels that they do not have the power to do anything about it – and the alcohol is used as an escape.

Because the effect of excessive marijuana use is not to be really present in the here and now, it can be associated with the root chakra, and tensions regarding money, home or work – though since it also might result in a sense of isolation and not being connected with others, it can also be seen as involving crown chakra tensions. It is important, again, to see what was going on in the person's life when the symptom began and what the person was unhappy about and wanting to escape from.

Because heroin is a Class A drug and so abuse of it is illegal, it points to crown chakra tensions in the person's relationship with their father or authority being a key to the dependency, as well as a sense of isolation and unhappiness in life, and the person being unhappy enough to consider dying.

With cocaine, in addition to possible crown chakra issues there may be solar plexus power and/or control issues, since its use inflates one's sense of personal power.

Since cigarette smoking is linked to problems with the heart and lungs, it represents tensions in the person's heart chakra and the area of relationships in their life, and some degree of discomfort about being loved and feeling loved.

Addison's Disease

Addison's disease is a condition brought about by the failure of the adrenal glands. The disease is characterized by weight loss, muscle weakness, fatigue, low blood pressure and sometimes darkening of the skin in both exposed and non-exposed parts of the body.

The adrenal glands are associated with the root chakra, as is the sense of fatigue, pointing to tensions in the areas of money, home and/or work (root chakra). Muscle weakness indicates solar plexus issues and the person not having a sense of their power, of not feeling 'I can.' Low blood pressure reflects something lacking in the area of relationships, and the darkening of the skin pigmentation points to crown chakra issues and a sense of separation or isolation.

Adenitis

Adenitis is inflammation of a lymph node or gland. Inflammation reflects anger, and the part of the body affected and the chakra associated with that part gives additional clues as to the tensions. At the level of the abdomen it reflects anger about sacral chakra issues – food or sex. When it occurs in the neck, it reflects anger that is not expressed, possibly because of insecurity (since the lymphatic system is associated with the root chakra).

Adenocarcinoma

Adenocarcinoma is a cancer that begins in glandular cells found in tissue that lines certain internal organs and makes and releases substances in the body, such as mucus, digestive juices or other fluids. Most cancers of the breast, pancreas, lung, prostate and colon are adenocarcinomas. Any cancer represents something held in, with the part of the body affected showing what it was that was not expressed. The location of the symptom and the chakra associated with that part of the body reflect the specific tension in the consciousness at the time in the person's life when the symptom began, with the understanding that if the symptom could have death as its logical conclusion, it began with a decision to die. The person was faced with a situation they found unacceptable and that they did not want to live with, and that situation would need to be resolved in order for the person to want to live. For further detail, see the part of the body or organ affected. See also Adenoma.

Adenoids (Tonsils)

Adenoids are one kind of tonsils, and when they are affected, they restrict the flow of air through the nose – pointing to difficulty letting in the love (air, heart chakra) at home (nose, root chakra) or from the mother. When the adenoids and/or tonsils are infected, this points to unexpressed anger (inflammation) affecting feeling not loved at home.

Adenoma

An adenoma is a benign tumour (-oma) of glandular origin. Adenomas can grow from many organs including the colon, adrenal glands, pituitary gland, thyroid and prostate. The area affected points to the chakra involved, and the specific tension in that area of the person's consciousness.

Any growth is considered to represent something held in and not expressed – so if it affects the colon, which is part of the elimination system, it is about root chakra tensions (money, home, job) and unexpressed insecurity or anger in that area, depending on which part of the colon is affected. The adrenal glands are related to the root chakra and issues of survival, fear and insecurity. Pituitary gland difficulties point to brow chakra tensions, and possible questions of being satisfied with being in a male or female body. Prostate difficulties in a man point to issues of trust with a woman.

Although these growths are benign, over time they may progress to become malignant, at which point they are called adenocarcinomas. Though benign, they have the potential to cause serious health complications by compressing other structures and by producing large amounts of hormones in an unregulated and non-retroactive manner, an anomaly called paraneoplastic syndrome. If they become malignant (life-threatening), then from the point of view that everything begins in the consciousness, the person affected has made the decision to die, being so unhappy about a situation that they have decided that they do not want to face life with that situation. Their healing would then have to involve not only releasing the symptom, but also resolving the situation they have been so unhappy about.

Adhesions

Adhesions are bands of scar-like tissue that form between two surfaces inside the body and cause them to stick together, usually after a surgical procedure. The adhesions can affect the female reproductive organs (ovaries, Fallopian tubes), the bowel, the area around the heart, the spine and the hands. They can cause a range of problems including infertility, painful intercourse, pelvic pain and bowel obstruction or blockage, reflecting tension in the consciousness in the root chakra, sacral chakra and heart chakra. Adhesions point to difficulties with a sexual partner at home and ambivalence about having a child at that time, or in that situation.

Adrenal Glands

The adrenal glands are located at the level of the solar plexus chakra, though they are related to the root chakra because they are triggered by fear or a threat to survival. Then, the hormones secreted can trigger either solar plexus functions (fight) or root chakra functions (flight). Problems with the adrenals therefore point to strong tensions in the root chakra parts of the person's life – money, home, work and/or the person's relationship with their mother.

The adrenal glands can also control kidney functions, pointing to the person's sense of not having the power or ability to deal with the unhappy situation they are in.

ADHD (Attention Deficit Hyperactivity Disorder) – See Hyperactivity

Aerophagia

Aerophagia is a repetitive pattern of swallowing or ingesting air and belching. It's normal to swallow a little air, but with aerophagia the amount of swallowed air is so large it can cause abdominal bloating, stomach pain and flatulence. It is sometimes due to nervousness or anxiety or is a symptom of hysteria. The symptom points to tensions in the solar plexus chakra and root chakra, and reflects insecurity about the person's power to do something about an unhappy situation.

Agoraphobia

In With panic disorder and agoraphobia, a person has attacks of intense fear and anxiety. There is also a fear of being in places from where it is hard to escape, or where help might not be available.

Agoraphobia usually involves fear of crowds, of bridges or of being outside alone. It is clearly associated with tension in the root chakra, and seeing through an emotional perceptual filter of fear. The person affected can look at what was happening in their life when the symptom began, in terms of root chakra parts of the consciousness – money, home, job, mother – to identify the situation they originally responded to with fear.

Because a sense of isolation is implied, it is important to look at crown chakra issues as well – tensions with the father and/or authority, and/or a sense of separation from someone close at the time the symptom began.

AIDS

AIDS (acquired immune deficiency syndrome) is the final stage of HIV, which causes severe damage to the immune system. Since that is related to the thymus gland, associated with the heart chakra, the symptom is associated with the person's perceptions of love. The person affected does not feel loved, either because of the use of socially unacceptable drugs, or their sexual preference, or the nature of the society in which they live.

During the initial infection a person may experience a brief period of influenza-like illness, and this also points to tensions in the heart chakra and thus is to do with the person's perceptions of love, tensions with someone close to their heart and not feeling loved.

In the case of children born to parents who are HIV positive, they do not feel the love connection with the parent affected.

Airsickness

Common signs and symptoms of airsickness include nausea and vomiting, which reflect a sense of losing control, as well as vertigo, dizziness, difficulty concentrating, confusion, drowsiness and increased fatigue, all pointing to root chakra tensions, insecurity and not feeling safe.

Airsickness can also cause headaches and reflect crown chakra tensions and a sense of isolation.

Alcoholism

Looking at the possible long-term effects of the abuse of substances can provide a clue to the chakra involved. If it is the liver that is affected, which is usual with alcohol abuse, then the solar plexus chakra is involved, and the issues are of power, control or freedom. The person is unhappy about something happening in their life, and does not have a sense that they have the power to do anything about it – and the alcohol is used as an escape.

The person affected is dealing with an addictive personality, which may manifest as addictions to other substances, or to a relationship in which they feel dependent on another person.

Allergic Rhinitis

Common symptoms of rhinitis are a stuffy nose, runny nose and post-nasal drip. The most common kind of rhinitis is allergic rhinitis, which is usually triggered by airborne allergens such as pollen.

Because it is the nose that has been affected, the symptom is related to tensions in the root chakra and, often, the person's relationship with their mother, and because it involves taking in air (love, associated with the heart chakra) through the nose, it can be related to difficulty letting in love from the mother, or difficulty letting in the love at home.

The symptom also points to insecurity or fear as a perceptual filter.

Allergic rhinitis may cause additional symptoms, such as sneezing and nasal itching, coughing (also associated with the heart chakra, pushing away the love, being angry at someone close to the person's heart), headache (connected with the crown chakra, a sense of separation/isolation), fatigue and cognitive impairment; not thinking clearly (both root chakra tensions). The allergens may also affect the eyes, causing watery, reddened or itchy eyes and puffiness around the area, which makes it look like the person is crying and indicates that the person is finding it difficult to look at something happening in their life.

Allergies

Allergies are sensitivities to normally harmless substances – and it is the effect of the allergy, the part of the body or function affected, that shows which chakra is involved, and which particular sensitivity in the consciousness is being triggered.

If the nose is affected, the sensitivity is in the root chakra, and therefore the tension is in the parts of the consciousness associated with the root chakra – issues of security: money, home, work and the person's sense of connection with their mother.

Allergies to wheat products and milk products point specifically to tensions with the mother, regardless of the physical effects of those particular substances, though the effects can also point to specific tensions with the mother.

If the elimination system is affected, for example if the person has diarrhoea or constipation, again, the root chakra tensions discussed above are involved.

If symptoms of the allergies are experienced as tensions in the solar plexus, the person can look at anger or issues concerning power, control or freedom. Skin issues also point to solar plexus tensions, though here it is important to look at the part of the body affected by the skin issues. The face, for example, could point to sensitivities about the person's image, how they feel they look to others or, in the case of acne as a perceived allergy, keeping potential partners at a distance because of sensitivities about freedom or being themselves in personal or sexual relationships.

Allergies that affect breathing point to sensitivities in the area of the heart chakra and perceptions of love, while those that affect the throat point to sensitivities concerning communication or expressing oneself.

Headaches point to crown chakra issues, reflecting tensions with the person's father and/or with authority, and a sense of isolation or separation from someone.

Alopecia in Women

Alopecia means baldness, loss of hair from the head or body. Whether it is only on the head or involving the entire body, it points to crown chakra tensions with the person's father/authority, and/or the person experiencing a sense of isolation or separation from someone, and not feeling connected with people around them.

Alzheimer's Disease

Alzheimer's disease is considered a form of dementia. The person has less and less contact with people around them, and they retreat more and more into their own world; this points to crown chakra and root chakra tensions. The person does not have their attention in the present moment and feels more and more isolated. They feel alone.

It may be possible to open the crown chakra by discussing the event that might have triggered their sense of isolation. See Amnesia, Anterograde amnesia.

Amblyopia – See Lazy Eye

Amenorrhoea

Amenorrhoea is the absence of a menstrual period in a woman of reproductive age. From the point of view that everything begins in the consciousness, it can arise from a decision not to have children, not to have to deal with the perceived inconvenience of monthly menstrual periods or not to want to function as an adult female, possibly because of a perceived disadvantage to being a woman.

AMI – See Acute Myocardial Infarction

Amnesia

There are two types of amnesia: anterograde and retrograde. Anterograde amnesia is the loss of long-term memory, the loss or impairment of the ability to form new memories through memorization. People may find themselves constantly forgetting a piece of information, people or events after a few seconds or minutes, because the data does not transfer successfully from their conscious short-term memory into permanent long-term memory. Primarily in older men, transient global amnesia can cause severe loss of memory for minutes or hours.

This type of amnesia is associated with root chakra tensions (since memory is associated with being present in the here and now), and possibly with the crown chakra and a sense of isolation and separation from someone, since when this chakra is closed the person is in his or her own world and not feeling connected with what is happening around them.

Retrograde amnesia is the loss of pre-existing memories to conscious recollection, beyond an ordinary degree of forgetfulness. This type of amnesia first targets the patient's most recent memories. The person may be able to memorize new things that occur after the onset of amnesia (unlike in anterograde amnesia), but is unable to recall some or all of their life or identity prior to the onset.

This type of amnesia is associated with the solar plexus chakra, since this chakra is connected with the mental body as well as the person's sense of identity. The memories still exist at the level of the spirit, or what the Western traditions know as the subconscious or unconscious, and are available through processes such as hypnosis that can bypass the normal mental processes. The trigger to repress the memory might have been an emotional shock. The emotional body and the person's willingness to feel their emotions is related to the sacral chakra. With an emotional shock, the person can decide to retreat inward to their mental body.

Amoeba Infection

Amoeba infection is a gastrointestinal parasitical infection that may or may not involve actual symptoms and can remain latent in an infected person for several years. Symptoms can range from mild diarrhoea to dysentery with blood and mucus in the stool. The symptoms in the elimination system indicate root chakra tensions about money, home and work, and possibly about not feeling safe at home; and if the liver is also affected, this reflects solar plexus tension and anger about root chakra issues. If the parasite reaches the bloodstream it can spread through the body, most frequently ending up in the liver, where it causes amoebic liver abscesses, which reflect anger.

As with any symptom, it is important to consider what was happening in the person's life at the time the symptoms manifested or were diagnosed.

Amoebiasis (Amoebic Dysentery)

The symptoms of amoebiasis can include loose stools, stomach pain and stomach cramping, reflecting tensions in the solar plexus chakra (anger) and in the root chakra (insecurity, fear). Amoebic dysentery is a severe form of amoebiasis that causes stomach pain, bloody stools and fever; it reflects anger and not feeling safe at home. If the liver is affected, this reflects anger, and symptoms in other parts of the body, such as the lungs or brain, reflect heart chakra tensions with someone close, and a sense of separation or isolation.

Amyotrophic Lateral Sclerosis (ALS)

Amyotrophic lateral sclerosis (ALS) – also known as motor neurone disease or Lou Gehrig's disease – is a debilitating disease characterized by rapidly progressive weakness, muscle atrophy, muscle spasticity, difficulty speaking, difficulty swallowing and decline in breathing ability. The muscle weakness and atrophy is throughout the body, and is caused by degeneration of the upper and lower motor neurons. Unable to function, the muscles weaken and atrophy.

As a neurological problem, this symptom points to crown chakra tensions and a sense of separation from someone and/or difficulties with authority – and fact the that the muscles are affected indicates that there are solar plexus issues such as the person not owning their power. The person by their way of thinking is making him or herself helpless, feeling that there is nothing they can do in a situation in their life that they are unhappy about. Breathing difficulties point to heart chakra tensions with someone close, who might be the 'authority figure' in the person's life.

Anaemia

Anaemia is a decrease in the number of red blood cells, or a lower than normal quantity of haemoglobin in the blood. Since this affects the blood's ability to carry oxygen to the various parts of the body, this reflects heart chakra tension with someone close, and the person's difficulty in allowing him or herself to be nourished by the love around them.

Andropause

As men get older, the level of testosterone in the body and production of sperm gradually becomes lower, and they experience physical and psychological symptoms as a result. Although symptoms may vary from person to person, common symptoms in men going through andropause include low sex drive, difficulties getting erections or erections that are not as strong as usual, lack of energy, depression, irritability and mood swings, loss of strength or muscle mass, increased body fat and hot flushes. Complications may include an increased risk of cardiovascular problems and osteoporosis (brittle bones). The symptoms point to a decrease in the activity of the sacral chakra, and tensions (insecurity) in the root chakra, possibly tensions at home. Some consider andropause to be a male menopause.

Aneurism (Aneurysm)

An aneurism is a localized, blood-filled balloon-like bulge in the wall of a blood vessel. Aneurisms commonly occur in arteries at the base of the brain or as aortic aneurisms, in the main artery carrying blood from the left ventricle of the heart.

Because aneurism involves blood, it is associated with the heart chakra and therefore tension with someone close to the person's heart; if the brain is affected, this reflects crown chakra tensions and a sense of separation from someone close to the person's heart.

Angina Pectoris

Angina pectoris, commonly known simply as angina, is chest pain due to a lack of blood, thus a lack of oxygen supply to and waste removal from the heart muscle, generally due to an obstruction or spasm of the coronary arteries (the heart's blood vessels). The symptoms point to tensions with someone close to the person's heart – a partner, parent, brother or sister, son or daughter. The tension is such that the person affected does not want to live with the situation in their life as it is.

Angioedema

Angioedema is a swelling that may accompany hives but occurs deeper in the skin. It is a swelling of the hands and feet, as well as the lips or eyelids. Hives is an irritation, and the part of the body and the function affected point to specific tensions in terms of what the person may be feeling irritated about. Thus, swelling in the feet reflects root chakra tensions and the person giving him or herself reasons to stay in the situation they find irritating; in the hands it indicates that the person is not allowing him or herself the fulfilment of receiving what they have asked for, or not wanting to touch others. Irritation and swelling of the lips may affect speech, and thus reflect the person not communicating what they feel irritated about, and if the eyes are affected, the person is not wanting to look at certain issues in their life that they find irritating. See also Hives.

Ankles

Anything affecting the ankles is related to root chakra tensions about money, home, work or the mother, and the effect of the symptoms (such as not being able to walk or stand) gives additional clues to the inner decision related to the symptom, when described from the point of view that the person created it. Thus, rather than saying the person cannot walk, we can say that they have been giving themselves reasons to stay in an unhappy situation, and keeping themselves from walking away. Difficulty standing reflects the person not standing on his or her own two feet, in a metaphoric sense – feeling insecure.

In right-handed people, the right ankle is seen as the male or the will ankle, and represents tensions about questions of trust in a man, or not trusting one's will, while the left ankle is seen as the female or emotional ankle, and represents tensions about not trusting a woman, or having been shaken to the foundations of one's emotional being.

The symptom can represent the person not putting their foot down; in a metaphorical sense, avoiding insisting on something; and if crutches are needed, the person has been soliciting support, needing others to agree with their point of view in terms of what they feel they must do.

Ankylosing Spondylitis

Ankylosing spondylitis is a form of spondyloarthritis, a chronic inflammatory arthritis. It mainly affects joints in the spine and the sacroiliac joint in the pelvis, and can cause eventual fusion of the spine. This points to tensions in the root chakra, and therefore tensions in the home or with the person's sense of connection with their mother as a nourishing energy. Insecurity and fear is a perceptual filter. As with any symptom, it is important to consider what was happening in the person's life at the time the symptom began. When it happens with a child, it can reflect a reaction to what was happening in the consciousness of the mother in relation to the child at that time.

Anorectal Bleeding

The most frequent causes of rectal bleeding are haemorrhoids, fissures and polyps. Diagnoses associated with difficulty in passing stool can range from constipation to faecal incontinence. In general, rectal bleeding is associated with not feeling safe at home. In the case of haemorrhoids, there may be a fear of losing something, and polyps or tumours in the colon represent something held in and not expressed concerning the root chakra parts of the person's consciousness – money, home, job. Depending on the location of the tumour in the colon, the emotional perceptual filter might be insecurity, or anger about root chakra issues. Tensions about the home could be about the family environment at home.

Anorexia Nervosa

Anorexia nervosa is an eating disorder characterized by extreme food restriction and irrational fear of gaining weight, as well as a distorted body self-perception. While it is considered an eating disorder, the chakra most involved is the solar plexus chakra, and the person is dealing with control issues overriding what their bodies are asking for. The person has turned off their sacral chakra. The extreme fear of gaining weight also points to root chakra tensions and not allowing oneself to be nourished.

Anorgasmia (Coughlan's Syndrome)

Anorgasmia, or Coughlan's syndrome, is a type of sexual dysfunction in which a person does not achieve orgasm, even with adequate stimulation. There may be sacral chakra tension, or ambivalence concerning sexual activity, though the root chakra is also often involved, reflecting the person feeling tensions with their partner and not feeling safe with their partner or comfortable letting go into the orgasm. The symptom is far more common in women than in men.

Anosmia

Anosmia is the loss of the sense of smell and is associated with tensions in the root chakra, and thus in the parts of the person's consciousness associated with issues of security (money, home, job), and also the person's sense of a lack of connection with their mother, and of not feeling nourished by their mother. When there is a loss of the sense of smell, the person is seeing the world through an emotional perceptual filter of insecurity or fear.

Antiphospholipid Syndrome

Antiphospholipid syndrome provokes blood clots in both arteries and veins, as well as pregnancy-related complications. It can stimulate organ failure. As a blood disorder, it relates to tensions in the heart chakra and thus the area of relationships, and since it is known to affect pregnancy, it can represent relational problems that give the person reasons not to want to bring a child into the world at that time, and which are possibly severe enough for the person to decide they would prefer to die rather than continue life with the unhappy situation as it is.

Anus

Anything affecting the anus of a person points to tensions in their root chakra concerning money, home, work or not feeling nourished by their mother, and not feeling safe at home. The person is seeing the world through an emotional perceptual filter of insecurity or fear.

Anxiety

Anxiety reflects tension in the root chakra. See what was happening in the person's life at the time when the anxiety began, in terms of the root chakra parts of the person's life – money, home, job, mother. What situation was it that the person responded to with insecurity or fear that has not been resolved, and has become a perceptual filter colouring the person's view of other things with fear?

Aortic Sclerosis

Sometimes calcium accumulates on the aortic valve, and the valve thickens, but the thickening does not interfere with blood flow through the valve. This disorder is called aortic sclerosis. About one out of four people over the age of sixty-five are said to have this disorder. Aortic sclerosis does not cause symptoms but may cause a soft heart murmur that can be heard by a doctor through a stethoscope. Aortic sclerosis may not make a person feel any different, but it increases the risk of a heart attack and death, and it points to heart chakra tensions, interfering with perceptions of love.

Aortic Stenosis

Aortic stenosis is the abnormal narrowing of the aortic valve. Symptoms include breathlessness, fainting, coughing at night and pains in the chest. Any symptom affecting the lungs or heart reflects heart chakra tensions with someone close, and fainting points to root chakra tensions. Thus, this symptom points to tensions with someone close and to not feeling the love at home.

Aphasia

Aphasia is a disorder caused by damage to the parts of the brain that control language. It can make it hard for the person to read, write and say what they mean to say. It reflects tension in the crown chakra, and therefore with the father and/or authority, and inhibited speech related to those tensions. There is difficulty communicating, for fear that what the person would like to express might not be okay with authority, or whomever the person perceives as authority.

Aphonia

Aphonia is the inability to produce voice. The person has shut their throat chakra and has been avoiding communicating about something important to them.

Aphthous Ulcer – See Canker Sores

Apnoea

'Apnoea' is the term used for when a person stops breathing. In sleep apnoea, the person stops breathing when they are asleep. Since both breathing and the element of air are associated with the heart chakra, a person's relationship with air reflects their relationship with love. Thus, in apnoea, the person is not allowing him or herself to let love in. Looking at what was happening in the person's life when this began can provide a clue to the situation the person responded to by feeling not loved, and so stopping the flow of love in their life.

Appendicitis

Appendicitis is a condition characterized by inflammation of the appendix. Because it is an inflammation, it can be associated with anger. Because the appendix is located on the right (will) side of the sacral chakra, the chakra that deals with the body asking for what it wants and needs in terms of food and sex, this symptom may reflect anger about the conflict between the person's will and what their body is asking for. While the appendix, going by its location, might seem to point to issues of food, or root chakra issues (because it affects the elimination system), it is interesting to notice the frequency with which this symptom occurs in adolescents, who are going through a sexual awakening; it could thus also point to insecurity or inner conflict about what the body is asking for in terms of food or sex, possibly because of confusing social values and attitudes in these areas.

Appetite

Appetite is associated with the sacral chakra, which represents the messages from the body to the person inside the body about what it wants or needs in terms of food and/or sex. Symptoms affecting the person's appetite can thus reflect tensions in these areas.

Arginase Deficiency

Arginase deficiency is a disorder that is considered to be inherited, which causes the amino acid arginine (a building block of proteins) and ammonia to accumulate gradually in the blood. Ammonia, which is formed when proteins are broken down in the body, is toxic if levels become too high. Toxins in the blood point to difficult emotions interfering with perceptions of love. The nervous system is especially sensitive to the effects of excess ammonia, and this points to crown chakra tensions with the father or authority, and/or a sense of isolation.

The symptom most often appears as stiffness, especially in the legs, caused by abnormal tensing of the muscles (spasticity). This reflects root chakra tensions (insecurity) and a sense of dependency (not standing on one's own two feet). Vomiting would also point to anger or a sense of losing control or going out of control. Other symptoms may include slower than normal growth and development (reluctance to grow up), intellectual disability, seizures, tremor and difficulty with balance and coordination (ataxia). This all reflects root chakra and crown chakra tensions, possible tensions between the parents and/or difficulty dealing with tensions at home.

Arms

The arms are controlled by the throat chakra, which is, among other things, about expressing goals; the arms represent the person reaching for their goals. In a right-handed person, the right arm represents the will arm and going for what they want, and the left arm represents the emotional arm and going for what makes them happy.

If the arms are immobilized, or if that could be the logical conclusion of the symptom if it were allowed to advance, and from the point of view that we each create our reality, then rather than saying that the person cannot use his/her arm, we could say that the person is keeping him or herself from reaching for something. The person had a specific goal at the time the symptom began, but has been talking to him or herself in a way that discourages them from going for that goal.

Arrhythmia

An arrhythmia is an irregular heartbeat. When symptoms of an arrhythmia occur, they may include palpitations, pounding in the chest, shortness of breath, chest discomfort, weakness or fatigue. Any symptoms involving the heart or breathing reflect tensions with someone close. Dizziness or feeling light-headed, or fainting, reflect root chakra tensions and thus tensions with someone at home.

Arterial Thrombosis

Arterial thrombosis is a blood clot that develops in an artery. It can obstruct the flow of blood to major organs, resulting in conditions such as heart attack – when the blood flow to the heart is affected; stroke – when the blood flow to the brain is affected; and/or peripheral arterial disease (PAD), also known as peripheral vascular disease (PVD) – when the blood flow in the legs is affected. Any symptom affecting the blood and/or heart reflects heart chakra tension with someone close. If the brain is affected, it reflects crown chakra tensions and a sense of separation from someone. If the legs are affected by this symptom, it reflects tension with someone close at home.

Arteries

The blood circulatory system is related to the heart chakra and thus the area of relationships and the person's perceptions of love. The arteries carry blood from the heart to the rest of the body, carrying nutrients and oxygen. So difficulties with the arteries reflect the person not allowing him or herself to feel nourished by the love around them.

If the symptom could eventually result in a heart attack, it reflects tensions with someone close to the person's heart – a partner, parent, sibling or child. If a specific part of the body is affected by the symptom, it points to specific tensions and decisions the person made at the time the symptom began or was discovered.

Arteriosclerosis

Hardening of the arteries occurs when fat, cholesterol and other substances build up in the walls of arteries and form hard structures called plaques. The blockage starves tissues of blood and oxygen, which can result in heart attack and stroke.

The symptom is related to the heart chakra and tensions with someone close to the person's heart – partner, parent, sibling or child. The person experiencing the symptom does not feel loved. They have difficulty allowing in the love from someone close.

Arthritis

Arthritis is a form of joint disorder that involves inflammation of one or more joints. The major complaint by individuals who have arthritis is joint pain.

In general, the skeletal system is related to the root chakra, but here, if the entire body is not affected, it is important to consider the affected part of the body. See the particular part affected for more detailed explanations.

Inflammation implies anger, and the effect of the symptom is immobility. Thus, the person is angry about their situation, and is immobilizing themselves through insecurity. If it is the hands that are affected, the person is keeping themselves from having what they have asked for, even though the solution may be available.

Asperger's Syndrome

Asperger's syndrome is a form of autism that is characterized by difficulties in social interaction, along with restricted and repetitive patterns of behaviour and interests. Physical clumsiness is frequently reported.

Autism is related to the crown chakra and the person's sense of connection with the father and authority. If the crown chakra is closed, the person experiences a sense of isolation, living in their own closed world with difficulty connecting with others, and not feeling the love around them. The repetitive patterns of behaviour point to tensions in the solar plexus chakra and issues of control, as well as tensions in the root chakra and a sense of insecurity or fear.

The physical clumsiness with this condition can also point to tensions in the root chakra, and a possible lack of connection with the mother as well, though this may be related to the extreme sense of isolation caused by the closed crown chakra.

As with any symptom, it is important to consider what was going on in the person's life when the symptom began, in terms of their sense of connection with their parents.

Asphyxia

Asphyxia is a lack of oxygen or excess of carbon dioxide in the body, usually caused by interruption of breathing, which causes unconsciousness. Because air is the element associated with the heart chakra, a person's relationship with air is said to reflect their relationship with love. Thus, with asphyxia, the person is having difficulty letting in the love. They are feeling not loved.

Asthenia

Asthenia is a condition of lack or loss of strength and energy; weakness. Generally, lack of strength is related to the muscles and therefore the solar plexus chakra, and the person not owning their power, making themselves helpless in the way they have been talking to themselves ('I can't...') Lack of energy also reflects root chakra tensions and insecurity, possibly not feeling safe at home. If the initial causes are neurological, as with multiple sclerosis, this can combine with crown chakra issues and the person can be described as not standing up to authority and making him or herself helpless before authority.

Asthma

Asthma is caused by inflammation in the airways, which makes the airways in the lungs swell and narrow. This reduces the amount of air that can pass by, leading to wheezing, shortness of breath, chest tightness and coughing.

The lungs are related to the heart chakra. A person's relationship with air reflects their relationship with love. Difficulty breathing in can be equated with difficulty letting in the love, and difficulty breathing out can relate to difficulty expressing love. Because the airways are irritated, it is important to consider what was happening in the person's life at the time the symptom began or was triggered, and to understand what it was the person felt irritated about; this would have affected their perceptions of feeling loved.

Astigmatism

Astigmatism is a distortion of the visual field. If it affects the will eye (the right eye in right-handed people), it indicates that the person has a distorted view of what they want. If it affects the other eye, the emotional eye, the person has a distorted sense of what they feel. If they are asked what they want or how they feel about a situation, they will think of something that is evident to them, but will decide that it is inappropriate, and express instead what they think they should want or feel. This is a distortion and this is why their vision is distorted on the physical level and that they see shapes distorted. Their vision shows them that this is a distortion.

The person is trying to fit in with values that are not theirs, in a situation where they feel that their true values and feelings are inappropriate or might create a perceived threat. If the person is no longer in the situation in which they made the decision that it is not okay to be themselves, they need to own their power and their right to be who they are (which is connected with the solar plexus chakra) and live their freedom and their truth.

Ataxia

Ataxia is a neurological symptom consisting of a lack of voluntary coordination of muscle movements, as in walking. Because the nervous system is affected, it reflects crown chakra tensions with authority or the father, and the effect of the symptom can reflect tension in other chakras. For example, if walking is affected, this means there is also tension in the root chakra, reflecting insecurity about standing up to authority. From the point of view that we each create our reality, the person has been keeping him or herself from walking, giving him or herself reasons to stay in an unhappy situation, when they would really like to walk away.

Athlete's Foot

Athlete's foot is a fungal infection of the skin that causes scaling, flaking and itching in the affected areas. Because it affects the feet, it can be related to the root chakra and the parts of the person's consciousness related to security and those things that represent security – money, home, work – and since it is a fungus, it can be described as 'gnawing away' in the person's consciousness, some constant background tension in the person's consciousness about security, possibly not feeling safe at home.

Atrophy

Atrophy is a wasting or decrease in the size of a body organ, tissue or part owing to disease, injury or lack of use.

To get a sense of the inner cause, see the particular part of the body affected, and/or the function affected. Thus, atrophy of the ovaries, for example, would point to tensions in the consciousness about sexuality or having children, since those would be the functions affected. Atrophy of the legs would point to the root chakra tensions concerning money, home, job, mother and keeping oneself from standing on one's own two feet, metaphorically.

Attention Deficit Hyperactivity Disorder (ADHD) – See Hyperactivity

Autism

Autism is related to the crown chakra and the person's sense of connection with their father and authority. When this is closed, the person experiences a sense of isolation, living in their own closed world with difficulties connecting with others, and not feeling the love around them.

As with any symptom, it is important to see what was going on in the person's life when the symptom began in terms of their sense of connection with their parents.

Autoimmune Disorders

Autoimmune disorders refer to a variety of symptoms said to be the result of a weakened immune system. To understand the inner cause of these symptoms, see the part of the body and/or the function affected. Because the immune system is related to the functions of the thymus gland, associated with the heart chakra, it can be said that this symptom is the result of tensions with someone close to the person's heart – a parent, partner, sibling or child.

Back Pain

If it is the entire back that hurts, it represents root chakra tensions in the consciousness – tensions about the parts of the person's life related to security (money, home, job, mother).

If it is a specific part of the back, the chakra closest to that part points to the specific tensions in the consciousness.

The sacral area (base of the spine) points to root chakra tensions, as described above, and insecurity or fear as a perceptual filter.

The lumbar area points to tensions in the sacral chakra having to do with issues of sexuality, food or having children. It can also reflect unreleased tensions in the emotional body, with the person suppressing those emotions, particularly in combination with root chakra tensions and constipation.

The level of the solar plexus points to tensions concerning power, freedom and/or issues of control. It can point to anger not yet released.

The back of the heart chakra, between the shoulder blades, points to tensions in the, possibly a sense of betrayal by a loved one.

The back of the neck points to tensions due to emotions not expressed, or something not communicated – sometimes a sense of carrying a burden.

If the tension is on the will side of the chakra, it reflects a conflict of will in that area, and on the emotional side, an emotional conflict.

Bad Breath

Halitosis or bad breath occurs when noticeably unpleasant odours are exhaled in breathing. Because the heart chakra is associated with the element of air, and the effect of the symptom is to keep others at a distance, this symptom is about not letting others get close. The person can be very loving, though perhaps not comfortable with feeling loved or letting in the love.

Balance

While the sense of balance is usually associated with the semicircular canals in the ear, it is related to the root chakra and being fully present in the physical body. See what was happening in the root chakra parts of the person's life (money, home, job, mother) at the time the sense of balance was affected, and the situation the person responded to with insecurity or fear.

Baldness

Baldness is related to tensions in the crown chakra and with the person's sense of connectedness with their father and/or authority.

Barlow's Syndrome (Mitral Valve Prolapse)

Barlow's syndrome is also known as mitral valve prolapse. The mitral valve between chambers of the heart malfunctions. Any condition affecting the heart reflects heart chakra tension with someone close. Palpitations and chest pain as symptoms also reflect heart chakra tensions. Symptoms like fatigue and anxiety point to root chakra tensions at home. Other symptoms – migraine headaches and, rarely, stroke – point to crown chakra tensions and a sense of isolation and separation from someone close.

Basedow's Disease – See Hyperthyroidism

Bed-Wetting

Bed-wetting is related to the root chakra and the person not feeling safe at home, and/or not feeling connected with their mother. Insecurity or fear is their perceptual filter.

Bee Stings – See Stings

Belching

While belching is a normal function, and can be related to what the person has been eating or drinking, or to swallowing air when eating or drinking, it can also be the result of excessive activity in the digestive process related to the solar plexus chakra, and thus related to issues of power, control and freedom. Tension in this chakra can be experienced in the consciousness as anger or an excessive need to control.

Bell's Palsy

The facial nerves control the muscles of the face, and when those are affected by facial paralysis, as in Bell's palsy, the result is an inability to control facial muscles on the affected side. This is related to tension in the brow chakra at the level of consciousness we know as the spirit, which the Western traditions know as the unconscious or subconscious. Because the effect can be seen as the person having received a strong slap in the face, see what was happening in the person's life at the time the symptom began, and how they may have felt themselves to be deeply insulted at that time.

The symptom can also be the result of a problem in one of the hemispheres of the brain, which would point to crown chakra issues and feeling separated from someone, and it can be seen how this condition and the one described above can both apply.

Benign Paroxysmal Positional Vertigo (BPPV)

Benign paroxysmal positional vertigo (BPPV) causes short episodes of intense dizziness (vertigo) or a spinning sensation when the person moves their head in certain directions.

It reflects root chakra tensions (insecurity or fear) about the parts of the person's life having to do with security (money, home, job) at the time the symptom began.

Benign Fasciculation Syndrome – See Twitch

Bipolar Disorder

Bipolar disorder, also known as manic-depressive disorder, is a state in which the person varies between manic periods when there are elevated energy levels and mood, and depressive episodes. This is related to the solar plexus chakra, and issues of power ('I can').

The person is facing a situation that they are unhappy with, but feel powerless to change, and are thus depressed about that. During the manic periods they spend time reaffirming their power until they again face the situation that they feel powerless to control, and then they return to the depressed state.

The situation is often an unhappy love story that the individual has not accepted for what it is.

Birth Defects

Birth defects (congenital disorders) are defined as symptoms existing at birth or before birth, or that develop during the first month of life. With the idea that symptoms on the physical level reflect tensions in the consciousness about something happening in the person's environment at the time the symptom began or was detected, the first consideration would be about when the symptom was actually detected. If it was apparent at birth, the symptom may have been the child's reaction to a difficult birth, or possibly it developed during pregnancy.

If the symptom began during pregnancy, it can represent the reaction of the child to what was going on in the consciousness of the parents about having the child at that time, and the child not feeling the contact, and therefore not feeling the love of its parents, since that was the environment to which it was responding.

If the symptom was diagnosed or discovered some time after birth, it is important to consider what was happening at the time it was diagnosed. For example, in the case of premature births, if the baby was in an incubator with no human contact for a period of time, and the symptom became apparent when he or she came out, it could be a reaction to the sense of isolation at that time, and thus tension in the crown chakra and a lack of a sense of contact with the father.

If the symptom was discovered later (possibly several years later), it is important to consider what was happening in the person's life at the time the symptom was discovered. The symptom on the physical level reflects decisions and tensions in the person's consciousness about what was happening in their life at that time, even when the medical view could be that it was something that had been there from birth.

For the specific birth defects, see the part of the body affected or function affected, and relate it to the above.

Blackheads

Blackheads are small bumps that appear on your skin due to clogged hair follicles. They are so called because the surface looks dark or black. They are a mild type of acne that usually forms on the face, but can also appear on the back, chest, neck, arms and shoulders.

Skin conditions reflect solar plexus tensions and therefore sensitivities about being oneself or about how one appears to others. When they appear on the face, they are designed to keep prospective partners at a distance, reflecting sensitivities about being oneself in relationships. Appearing on parts of the body usually kept covered reflects sensitivities about taking off one's clothes in the presence of another, and therefore sensitivities about intimate contact. The symptom on the chest and back reflects solar plexus tensions in the area of the heart chakra, which means sensitivities about freedom or being oneself in a relationship; and on the arms and shoulders, ambivalence about setting goals in the relationship due to considerations of power, control and freedom.

Bladder Problems

The bladder is related to the root chakra, and the parts of the person's consciousness having to do with security, survival and trust, and the parts of their life related to security (money, home, work), as well as the person's sense of connection with their mother as a source of security and nourishment. Bladder problems thus reflect tensions in one or more of these areas.

Bleeding

See the part of the body or the function affected in order to understand the inner cause of the symptom. For excessive bleeding, see also Haemorrhage.

Blindness

Described from the point of view that we each create our reality, when someone is blind, the person is keeping him or herself from seeing something, or avoiding looking at something. The type of blindness gives clues to the trigger in the person's consciousness that created the symptom.

The person is experiencing a sense of isolation and feeling that they have nothing to look forward to, and the conditions in their life at the time the symptom began can be examined to understand the reasons for the decision.

The blindness might be due to difficulties with the cornea or the retina, or cataracts, or glaucoma. See these particular organic symptoms in this listing for further details.

Blindness in just one eye can reflect not seeing the male or not seeing the female in their life, indicating a sense of separation from a man or a woman at the time the symptom began, with a possible sense that they will not connect with a male or a female in their life in the future.

Blisters

Blisters represent anger, and the specific part of the body affected and the function affected point to the inner cause of the symptom. For example, blisters on the tongue reflect unexpressed anger, since it can affect the person's speech. A blister on the eyelid that might affect the person's vision could represent anger keeping the person from seeing something related to a male or female, depending on whether it is their male or female eye, or difficulty looking at something contrary to what the person wants (their will eye) or what will make them happy (their emotional eye). Blisters affecting the sexual function point to anger about sexuality, or the person keeping him/herself from sexual activity because of anger.

Bloating

Bloating is any abnormal general swelling, or an increase in diameter of the abdominal area. The person feels a full and tight abdomen, possibly with abdominal pain; this points to solar plexus tensions about anger or excessive control. There may be chest pains or shortness of breath, pointing to heart chakra tensions with someone close.

Blood

In general, the blood is related to the heart chakra, and thus issues of relating or relationships – tensions concerning perceptions of love. Blood disorders point to tensions with someone close to the person's heart – a partner, parent, sibling or child – or decisions and beliefs affecting perceptions of love. See the specific symptoms to understand the inner cause as a response to what was happening in the person's life at the time the symptom began.

Blood Pressure

Blood pressure is related to the heart chakra, and therefore the area of relationships in a person's life. High blood pressure would be related to tensions with someone close. Low blood pressure could point to lack of energy or lack of motivation in the situation with someone close to the person's heart – a parent, partner, sibling or child.

Blood Sugar

Blood sugar refers to the amount of glucose in the blood, and relates to the amount of 'sweetness' the person experiences in their life. See Diabetes for excessive blood sugar, and see Hypoglycaemia for low blood sugar.

Body Hair – See Hirsutism

Body Odour

According to many societal norms, body odour is considered unpleasant, though this is not a universal perception. Where it is seen as a problem, it has the effect of keeping others away, particularly in the areas of social contact (heart chakra) or sexual contact (sacral chakra), so it is the sensitivities in these areas that can be associated with unpleasant body odour. When the body odour can be related to the elimination system (excessive sweating, for example), root chakra tensions and insecurities may play a part. When sensitivities in these areas are resolved, the person can experience a shift in their consciousness that allows them to see the benefits of different habits of cleanliness and grooming.

Boils (Furuncles)

Boils represent anger, and the location of the boils points to what the anger is about, in terms of the parts of the body or the function affected. For example, boils on the tongue could indicate unexpressed anger, since this can affect the person's speech. A boil on the eyelid that might affect the person's vision could represent anger keeping the person from seeing something related to a male or female, depending on whether it is their male or female eye, or something contrary to what the person wants (their will eye) or what will make them happy (their emotional eye). Boils may occur in the hair follicles anywhere on the body but are most common on the face, neck, armpit, buttocks and thighs. Boils affecting the sexual function would point to anger about sexuality or the person keeping him or herself from having sex because of anger. On the buttocks and thighs they can reflect anger about root chakra issues, or anger at home.

Bone Marrow

Bone marrow is the flexible tissue found in the interior of bones. In humans, red blood cells are produced in the heads of long bones. Bone marrow is also a key component of the lymphatic system, producing the lymphocytes that support the body's immune system.

In general, the skeletal system is related to the root chakra, and the function of the bone marrow points to the production of red blood cells that take nourishment to the various parts of the body through the blood circulatory system, associated with the heart chakra.

Thus, the bone marrow represents heart chakra considerations in the region of the root chakra, or something about allowing oneself to be nourished by the love at home. Since the lymphatic system is also possibly involved, this points again to the root chakra, and the possibility of the person having had difficulty releasing difficult emotions regarding someone close to their heart at home.

Bone Spurs – See Osteophytosis

Bone Tumours

Bone tumours may be classified as 'primary tumours', which originate in the bones, or 'secondary tumours', which originate in other sites and spread (metastasize) to the skeleton. Carcinomas of the prostate, breasts, lungs, thyroid and kidneys are the primary carcinomas that most commonly metastasize to the bone; these all reflect various relational difficulties with someone at home.

Tumours represent something held in and not expressed, and the location of the tumour points to what has not been expressed. If the tumour is in a particular location, that location points to the inner cause. Similarly, the function that is affected, or that would be affected if the symptom were allowed to continue to its logical conclusion, also points to the inner cause when described from the point of view that the person created it. Thus, a bone tumour in the leg would point to root chakra tensions (insecurity or non-trust) held in and not expressed, and if the possible effect would be for the person not to be able to walk, the person has been keeping him or herself from walking – talking to themselves in a way that convinces them to stay in some unhappy situation.

If the tumour is secondary, that is, a metastasis of a tumour elsewhere in the body, root chakra considerations would be reflected in addition to the message of the primary tumour. If the primary tumour was in the breast or lung, for example, it would reflect tension in the area of relationships, with someone close to the person's heart, and if the metastasis appeared later in the bone, it would reflect tensions with someone at home, someone the person is living with.

If the tumour is malignant, and death could be the logical conclusion of the symptom, the person has decided that the situation they are in is unacceptable, and that they do not want to face life with that situation in it. Their healing, then, must also involve resolving that unhappy situation.

Bones

When it is the entire skeleton that is affected, as with systemic arthritis or osteoporosis, the skeletal system is related to the root chakra. Otherwise, when the bones are affected in a particular part of the body, that part or the function affected would point to the inner cause, with the root chakra as a possible contributing cause. Thus, a broken right arm in a right-handed person could point to something about insecurity or broken trust (root chakra) about reaching for goals (arms) concerned with what the person wants (will side).

Bowels

In human anatomy, the intestine (or bowel) is the segment of the gastroin-testinal tract extending from the stomach to the anus and consists of two segments, the small intestine and the large intestine. Generally, the small intestine is related to the process of assimilation, and associated with the second (sacral) chakra, and the person's relationship with food and assim-ilating its nutrients, or being nourished by the food. The large intestine, the colon, is related more specifically to the root chakra and the process of elimination. Part of the colon crosses the solar plexus chakra, and when this part, the transverse colon, is affected, it represents a combination of conditions involving the solar plexus chakra and the root chakra – thus, possible anger about root chakra issues, which are issues about money, home and work.

Since any part of this system could be related to eventual elimination, any symptoms here reflect tension about root chakra issues in the person's life. If there is physical discomfort, see which chakra is closest to the phys-ical sensation of tension (if it is the second or third chakra) and consider tensions in that part of the person's consciousness in relation to root chakra issues.

Bradycardia

Bradycardia is a slow heart rate, and it sometimes results in fainting, short-ness of breath and, if severe enough, death. It is associated with the heart chakra, and therefore the person's perceptions of love. The person is not feeling loved, or is not allowing him or herself to be nourished by the love around them. If it results in fainting, the person is going out of their body, letting go at the level of the root chakra and experiencing insecurity or fear as a perceptual filter, possibly about the relationship in question.

Brain, General

The brain is related to the crown chakra, which has to do with feeling either connected or isolated, and to the person's relationship with their father and/or authority. Symptoms affecting the brain therefore reflect tensions with the person's father or authority, or a reaction to a sense of separation from someone, creating a sense of isolation in the person's consciousness in response to something happening in their life at the time the symptom began. See other parts of the body or functions that may be affected for more details.

Brain Haemorrhage – See Stroke

Brain Tumour (Ganglioglioma)

Any tumour represents something held in and not expressed, and the part of the body affected shows what it is that was being held in or not expressed at the time the symptom began, in response to what was happening in the person's life at that time. Because it is the brain, the event at that time involved tension with the father or authority, or a sense of separation from someone close. Because the apparent logical conclusion of the symptom can be death, and working with the idea that everything begins in the consciousness, the person reacted to a situation they found unacceptable, and decided that they did not want to face life with that situation as it was. See other parts of the body or functions that may be affected for more details.

Breast Cancer

Cancer represents something held in and not expressed, and the part of the body affected shows what it was. With breast cancer, the closest chakra to the symptom is the heart chakra, and therefore the symptom represents tension concerning something that happened with someone close to the person's heart (partner, parent, sibling, child) at the time the symptom began. The apparent logical conclusion of the symptom shows something about the tension in the consciousness associated with the symptom. If one logical conclusion would be removal of the breast, and we think from the point of view that we each create our reality, the person has been cutting herself off from her femininity, manifesting more yang characteristics (hardness) than her natural state of balance, suppressing her yin characteristics (softness) because of the remaining tensions in her consciousness about what happened when the symptom began.

If we view death as an apparent logical conclusion, it reflects the person's decision to die, deciding that she does not want to face life with that unacceptable situation. The healing of the symptom therefore involves resolving the situation in some way. See also Breasts, below.

Breasts

The breasts are associated with the heart chakra, and symptoms affecting the breasts therefore reflect tension with someone close to the person's heart at the time the symptom began or was discovered. If the will breast is affected (right breast in a right-handed person), it represents something in a relationship that is different from what the person wants, and if it is the emotional breast, it represents an emotional reaction to what was happening in the relationship at the time the symptom began or was discovered.

Because the breasts represent the nourishing mother energy and femininity in general, if the symptom involves possible removal of the breast we should consider these aspects. In this case, from the point of view that we each create our reality, the person has been cutting herself off from her femininity, manifesting more yang characteristics (hardness) than her natural state of balance, suppressing her yin characteristics (softness), because of the remaining tensions in her consciousness about what happened when the symptom began.

Breathing

The lungs are related to the heart chakra, associated with the element of air. A person's relationship with air therefore reflects their relationship with love. Difficulty breathing in can be equated with difficulty letting in the love, and difficulty breathing out can relate to difficulty expressing love.

If there is difficulty breathing through the nose, which is related to the root chakra and the person's relationship with their mother, it reflects difficulty letting in the love from the mother, or difficulty letting in the love at home.

If the difficulty in breathing is due to tensions in the throat, it reflects tensions in the throat chakra affecting the flow of love – difficulty expressing emotions or difficulty communicating, which is resulting in difficulty letting in the love.

Bright's Disease

Bright's disease is the historical name given to a classification of kidney diseases that would be described in modern medicine as acute or chronic nephritis. It is typically identified by the presence of serum albumin (blood plasma protein) in the urine, and frequently accompanied by swelling and hypertension.

The kidneys are associated with the elimination system, and therefore with the root chakra, though they are located at the level of the solar plexus chakra. Symptoms involving the kidneys thus point to root chakra considerations at the level of the solar plexus or, in other words, insecurity about power. The person has a perceived lack of power. They are in an unhappy situation but feel that they are helpless to change it. They are making themselves helpless or dependent in their way of thinking, not owning their power.

The presence of blood plasma protein in the urine can also reflect a person not allowing themselves to be nourished by the love at home.

If there are kidney stones, the person experiences pain at the level of the kidneys, at the level of the solar plexus chakra, again pointing to tensions concerning their sense of insecurity about their power.

Bone loss associated with kidney disease points to other root chakra tensions, including a loss of a sense of solidity or stability, not feeling supported and insecurity as a perceptual filter.

Hypertension associated with kidney disease points to heart chakra issues – tensions with someone close like a partner, parent, sibling or child, and the person feeling powerless to change the situation.

Broken Bone

While the skeletal system as a whole is associated with the root chakra, a symptom affecting the bone in a particular part of the body can be read according to the part of the body affected, and the chakra associated with that part, as well as the perceived effect of the symptom, when described from the point of view that the person created it.

Bronchial Asthma – See Asthma

Bronchial Pneumonia

Bronchial pneumonia involves inflammation of the bronchial tubes due to infection. As with any kind of pneumonia, the symptoms include cough, rapid breathing, chest pain and shortness of breath. Symptoms affecting the lungs reflect tensions in the heart chakra, thus tensions with someone close to the person's heart – a parent, partner, sibling or child. The heart chakra is associated with the element of air, and a person's relationship with air reflects their relationship with love. Inflammation implies anger. Coughing is seen as the person pushing away the air, difficulty letting in the love from the person with whom there has been tension. When there is fever, it reflects anger. When headaches are involved, it reflects crown chakra tensions and a sense of separation from someone. Weakness would reflect a sense of powerlessness in the situation where there has been tension.

Bronchiectasis

Bronchiectasis is a condition caused by mucus blockage in which the lungs' airways are abnormally stretched and widened. Because the lungs are associated with the heart chakra and the person's perceptions of love, this symptom is related to difficulty letting love in, either because of an event the person responded to by not feeling loved by someone close, or else because of a closed crown chakra, reflecting a sense of separation from someone close or tensions with father/authority at the time the symptom began.

Bronchitis

Bronchitis is a cough, an inflammation of the mucous membranes of the bronchi, the airways that carry airflow from the trachea into the lungs. Because the lungs are associated with the heart chakra, and the element of air, a person's relationship with air reflects their relationship with love. The person is pushing away the air, pushing away the love, angry with someone close to his or her heart.

Brow Chakra Tensions

The brow chakra is associated with the deeper part of your consciousness, the spirit, known in Western traditions as the subconscious or unconscious. Tensions at this level that could result in brow chakra symptoms can include tensions about religion or spirituality (too many rules, spiritual addiction to an organization), or tensions about the inner senses commonly referred to as ESP, or spirit-to-spirit communication, if the person is not comfortable with those impressions. Deep tensions about disturbing events or a deep sense of insult might be held here if the person finds them difficult to deal with. Difficulty relating to the gender of the physical body could result in tensions at this level.

Bruises/Abrasions

See the part of the body affected and the chakra associated with that part of the body in order to get a sense of how the person felt 'bruised' or sore, annoyed in their consciousness in response to what was happening in their life when the symptom occurred. See also Ecchymoses.

Bruxism

Bruxism refers to excessive grinding of the teeth and/or excessive clenching of the jaw. The jaw is associated with the solar plexus chakra and the teeth with the root chakra. Thus, the symptom points to anger about the root chakra parts of the person's life – money, home, job, mother – at the time the symptom began.

Bubonic Plague

Bubonic plague is an infection of the lymph nodes. Symptoms include smooth, painful lymph gland swellings called buboes; these commonly occur in the groin, and reflect anger about root chakra tensions about home, although they may also occur in the armpits or neck, most often at the site of the infection (which is a bite or scratch). In these locations they reflect insecurity about expressing or communicating.

Pain may occur in the area before the swelling appears.

Other symptoms include chills and fever, reflecting anger about root chakra tensions; muscle pain, reflecting a feeling of being powerless; headache and seizures, reflecting crown chakra tensions with father/authority and a sense of isolation.

Bulimia

Bulimia nervosa is an eating disorder characterized by binge eating and purging, or consuming a large amount of food in a short amount of time followed by an attempt to rid oneself of the food consumed (purging), typically by vomiting, taking a laxative or diuretic and/or excessive exercise.

Since it is considered an eating disorder, it might mean the second (sacral) chakra, associated with food and sex, is overactive, though the compulsion to get rid of the food or its effects afterwards also points to control issues at the level of the solar plexus.

Bunions

A bunion is a deformity of the joint connecting the big toe to the foot. It reflects tensions in the consciousness in the root chakra, most likely in the person's relationship with their home, specifically not feeling safe at home.

Burns

Because the solar plexus chakra is associated with the element of fire, burns reflect anger, and the part of the body affected and its associated chakra provides additional details concerning the cause of the anger and/or the perceived effect.

Bursitis

Bursitis is the inflammation of one or more bursae (small sacs) of synovial fluid in the body. The bursae rest at the points where muscles and tendons slide across bone.

Inflammation points to anger, and the part of the body affected and its associated chakra give additional clues to the cause of the anger and/or the perceived effect. If one effect is immobility, for example, the person has been immobilizing him or herself in some way as a result of the anger that has been held in and not expressed.

Buttocks

The buttocks are the rear pelvic area of the human body, the sitting muscles, commonly referred to as the 'butt' or the 'behind'. They are associated with the root chakra, and with a person's relationship with security, or trust, and the parts of the person's life associated with security or trust – usually money, home and job. Thus, symptoms affecting the buttocks would reflect tension in the root chakra parts of the person's life, and the person seeing through an emotional perceptual filter of insecurity or fear. If only one side is affected, it reflects insecurity concerning what the person wants (will side) or what they feel (emotional side), or lack of trust with a male (male side) or a female (female side).

Calculus – See Tartar

Calluses

A callus is a toughened area of skin that has become relatively thick and hard in response to repeated friction, pressure or other irritation. Since repeated contact is required for this thickening, calluses are most often found on the feet because of the action of walking. They are generally not considered to be a problem or pathological, but may sometimes appear on areas considered unusual for them. In these cases, they may reflect insensitivity about something, and the location of the callus can provide more specific information as to what they reflect in terms of tensions in the consciousness.

Calluses on the hands of someone who is not involved in manual labour, for example, can reflect a lack of feeling with regard to allowing him or herself to fulfil a goal, or a reluctance to touch people. See Hands.

For more details, see the part of the body affected by the callus.

Cancer, General

Cancer represents something held in and not expressed; the part of the body affected and the associated chakra show what it is that has been held in and not expressed. It is a message from the person's higher self letting him or her know what they need to do differently in their life in order for them to return to their natural state of balance.

Lung cancer, for example, because of its association with the heart chakra, reflects tension with someone close to the person's heart (a partner, parent, brother or sister, son or daughter) and since the symptom can affect breathing, and the element of the heart chakra is air, the person's relationship with air reflects their relationship with love. The tension in their consciousness about something that happened in their life at the time the symptom began has been giving the person reasons not to feel loved by someone, and not to allow in the love from that person.

Regardless of the part of the body affected, the eventual logical conclusion of the symptom – death – shows that the person has decided that the situation they are in is unacceptable, and that they would rather die than continue with that situation in their life. For them to decide to live, they must resolve this tension or the situation so that they have something to look forward to, something to live for.

See the part of the body affected to understand more specifics about the inner cause and what it has been communicating to the person affected.

Cancer of the Ovaries – See Ovarian Cyst, Ovarian Cancer

Candida (Fungus)

Candida is a kind of yeast. Many species are harmless but other species, or a harmless species in the wrong location, can cause disease. Candida albicans can cause infections (candidiasis or thrush) in humans and other animals, especially in patients whose immune systems have been compromised, such as people with AIDS or HIV.

A fungus is something that eats, so someone affected by a yeast infection or a fungus can be said to have something eating away at them, in their consciousness. The part of the body affected can show what it is about. For example, a yeast infection in the genital area can be said to represent something eating away at the person, bothering them, about sex. The symptom would discourage them from sexual activity; so from the point of view that we each create our reality, the person is keeping him or herself from having sex. They want it, but have been giving themselves reasons not to have it.

If the symptom affects the root chakra, located at the level of the perineum, it can represent something eating away at their sense of security, bothering them about money, home, work or their connection with their mother, though if it discourages sexual contact, the insecurity can be about their sexuality.

A systemic candida infection affecting the skin could be seen as representing tensions in the person's solar plexus chakra, associated with the skin and which has to do with the person's feelings about their appearance, the face or image they show the world and their sense of freedom to be who they are. If others are discouraged from getting close, the person has been creating a sense of isolation; this also points to crown chakra tensions with father/authority.

Candidiasis (Thrush)

Candidiasis, also called thrush, is a yeast infection that can affect the skin of the vagina, the penis or the mouth, reflecting something about intimate contact bothering the person in the background of their consciousness. It may also infect the bloodstream, reflecting heart chakra tensions with someone close, or possibly internal organs such as the liver or spleen, reflecting background anger. See Candida, above.

Canker Sores

An aphthous ulcer, also known as a canker sore, is a type of ulcer that presents as a painful open sore inside the mouth or upper throat, and is characterized by a break in the mucous membrane. It is not considered contagious.

An ulcer is associated with anger; one affecting the mouth and throat represents anger unexpressed, and therefore tension in the throat chakra. Since the symptom itself can also indicate that the person tends to keep people at a distance, it can also represent the person isolating him or herself, because the ulcer is giving him or herself reasons to avoid social or sexual contact.

Carbuncle

A carbuncle is a skin infection that often involves a group of hair follicles. They may develop anywhere, but they are most common on the back and the nape of the neck. Infection or irritation points to anger, and the location gives an indication of additional considerations. For example, on the neck it can mean that the anger was not expressed. On the back, at the level of the heart chakra, it could reflect anger in a relationship. As always, the person needs to look at what was happening in their life at the time the symptom began.

Cardiovascular Disease

Any kind of cardiovascular disease (heart disease) reflects tension in the heart chakra, and therefore tension in the area of relationships with someone close to the person's heart.

Caries

Caries is the progressive destruction of any kind of bone structure, including the skull, ribs and other bones or the teeth. When it affects the teeth, it reflects insecurity and/or an erosion of trust at home, since the teeth are related to the root chakra. In other examples of caries, affecting the bone in other parts of the body, the part of the body affected and the chakra that is closest reflect more details about the erosion of trust in that area.

Carpal Tunnel Syndrome (Nerves in the Hand)

The area in your wrist where the nerve enters the hand is called the carpal tunnel. This tunnel is normally narrow, so any swelling can pinch the nerve and cause pain, numbness, tingling or weakness. This is carpal tunnel syndrome. It is a condition in which there is pressure on the median nerve – the nerve in the wrist that provides feeling and movement to the 'thumb side' of the hand (the palm, thumb, index finger, middle finger and thumb side of the ring finger). While many people believe that carpal tunnel syndrome is caused by making the same hand and wrist motion over and over, for example by typing on a computer, using a mouse or repeating movements while working or playing an instrument, the inner cause, the tension in the person's consciousness, reflects how the person feels about the situation they are in while making those repetitive movements. If it is their job, how does the person feel about doing that job?

The wrists and hands represent the person allowing themselves to have the fulfilment of what they want or of what will make them happy, depending on whether it is the will hand or the emotional hand, and each finger can represent a chakra. Thus, a right-handed person experiencing difficulties with the thumb on the right hand can be seen to be experiencing tensions in their consciousness related to letting themselves have what they want (or what will make them happy) in relation to root chakra parts of their life (money, home, job). Then, it is interesting to see how the symptom is related to something they are doing at work, and it raises the question of whether they are happy at work or would really prefer to be doing something different. The index finger would point to issues concerning the person allowing themselves to have what they want regarding food or sex, and the middle finger to solar plexus issues of power, control or freedom.

Carsickness – See Motion Sickness

Cataracts

A cataract is a clouding of the lens inside the eye, resulting in a decrease in vision. It is associated with the person having decided that they have nothing to look forward to, so it is important to consider what was happening in the person's life that stimulated that decision.

If the cataract is in the male eye (the right eye in right-handed people), it reflects a sense of separation from a male at that time, with the person deciding that they have nothing to look forward to regarding having a male in their life. If the female eye is affected, it reflects the person deciding they have nothing to look forward to regarding having a female in their life.

When both eyes have been affected, it points to the person making a general decision about having nothing to look forward to. The sense of isolation resulting from blindness points to crown chakra tensions and thus a sense of separation from someone.

Catatonia

Catatonia is a state of apparent unresponsiveness to external stimuli in a person who is apparently awake. There may or may not be physical immobility. The lack of response to external stimuli reflects crown chakra tension with father/authority or a state of isolation as a response to a sense of separation from someone close.

Cavities – See Caries

Celiac Disease – See Coeliac Disease

Cellulite

Cellulite is a term used to describe skin with a dimpled appearance, caused by fat deposits just below the surface of the skin. It generally appears on skin in the abdomen, lower limbs and the buttocks and hips, and because it usually occurs after puberty, it can be associated with how the person feels about their sexuality. From the point of view that we each create our reality, and because it is generally considered unattractive, it can be said that the person has been making him or herself unattractive because of sensitivities concerning sexuality, and therefore tensions in the sacral chakra. Because the legs are also usually affected, the symptom points to insecurity (tension in the root chakra) concerning sexuality.

When there is a part of the anatomy that the person is particularly self-conscious about, there is a concentration of attention in that area – and in this case, it is in the areas of the first two chakras. It can be interesting to consider why the person has been holding so much attention there.

Cephalea (Headache)

Pain in the head is associated with tension in the crown chakra, pointing to issues of isolation and separation, or tension with the father and/or authority, at the time the symptom began. See Headache.

Cerebral Ictus (Brain Haemorrhage) – See Stroke

Cerebral Palsy

Cerebral palsy is caused by injuries to or abnormalities of the brain. Most of these problems occur as the baby grows in the womb, but they can happen at any time during the first two years of life, while the baby's brain is still developing. Because it involves the brain, it is associated with the crown chakra, and tensions involving the person's sense of connection (or lack of it) with their father at the time the symptom began.

Cervical Cancer

The cervix, where this cancer starts, is the lower part of the uterus (womb) that opens out at the top of the vagina. Because it is located in the uterus, it can be associated with tensions in the sacral chakra and therefore issues about having a child, but this symptom is often found in women no longer of childbearing age; its location in these cases can also be thought of as being at the level of the root chakra, representing trust – and thus it also reflects a lack of trust with a man.

As with any cancer, cervical cancer represents something held in and not expressed, and the part of the body affected shows what this was. Looking at what was happening in the life of the person affected at the time the symptom began or was detected can give insights into the decisions creating it; we can look at it as the person deciding that the situation was unacceptable, and that she did not want to face life with this situation in it.

Cervix – See Cervical Cancer

Chest

Generally, any symptom in the chest area would be associated with tensions in the heart chakra, and therefore in the area of relationships in the person's life – specifically their relationship with someone close to their heart. That could be a partner, parent, sibling or child. The particular symptom and whether it was located on the will side or the emotional side would give further details about what was happening in the person's life at the time the symptom began, and the decisions the person made at that time in response to those conditions.

Chicken Pox

Chicken pox is a viral infection in which a person develops extremely itchy blisters all over the body. Most children with chicken pox have fever, headache and stomach ache before the rash appears; this points to issues of anger (solar plexus) and, since it is considered contagious, a sense of isolation (crown chakra tensions). From the point of view that we each create our reality, the person has been isolating him or herself. This, as well as the symptom of headaches, also points to crown chakra issues – possible tensions with father and/or authority.

Chills

This term can refer to feeling cold after exposure to a cold environment and also to an episode of shivering, accompanied by paleness and feeling cold. Chills may occur at the beginning of an infection and are usually associated with a fever. The fever points to a sense of anger, and the chills can be related to feeling 'left out in the cold' – feeling the lack of contact with someone close at the level of the heart chakra.

Chlamydia

Chlamydia infection is a sexually transmitted disease.

In men, symptoms may include a burning sensation during urination and discharge from the penis or rectum, reflecting root chakra tensions and therefore insecurity, likely about sexuality. There may be testicular tenderness or pain, reflecting tensions about sexuality.

In women, symptoms that may occur include a burning sensation during urination and rectal pain or discharge, reflecting root chakra tensions and thus insecurity, likely about sex. Painful sexual intercourse gives the person a reason to avoid sex. Liver inflammation as a symptom reflects anger. The Fallopian tubes may be affected as well, reflecting ambivalence about having children. See also Pelvic Inflammatory Disease (PID).

Choking

Choking is the blocking of the flow of air into the lungs. Choking prevents breathing, and because the element of air is associated with the heart chakra, it therefore reflects difficulty letting in the air – difficulty letting in the love from someone close.

Cholelithiasis – See Gall-Bladder Calculosis (Gallstones)

Cholera

Cholera is an infection of the small intestine that causes a large amount of watery diarrhoea.

Symptoms can include lethargy, low urine output and unusual sleepiness or tiredness, and these symptoms point to tensions in the root chakra (security, survival, trust). Nausea and vomiting reflect tension in the solar plexus chakra and the feeling of things going out of control. Lack of tears reflects unexpressed unhappiness about something happening in the person's life. It's no accident that this symptom occurs in parts of the world where people are dealing with survival issues and feeling they can do nothing about it.

Cholesterol – See Arteriosclerosis

Chronic Bronchitis – See Bronchitis

Chronic Fatigue Syndrome

Chronic fatigue syndrome refers to severe, continued tiredness that is not relieved by rest and is not directly caused by other medical conditions. This reflects tension in the root chakra, and thus the parts of the person's consciousness associated with money, home and job. The person can ask him or herself what they are 'tired of.'

Specific symptoms can point to specific causes:

- Forgetfulness and concentration problems, as well as confusion, point to tensions in the root chakra parts of the person's life, including money, home, job and/or mother.
- Joint pain but no swelling or redness indicate root chakra tensions; immobilizing oneself because of insecurity.
- Headaches – crown chakra tensions with father and authority, and/or a sense of separation or isolation.
- Irritability – anger triggered by insecurity – tensions in the solar plexus and root chakras.
- Mild fever (no more than 101 degrees F/38 degrees C) – anger.
- Muscle aches and/or muscle weakness – solar plexus chakra tensions: not owning one's power; feeling powerless in an unhappy situation. Immobilizing oneself with a perceived lack of power ('I can't.')
- Sore throat – unexpressed anger
- Sore lymph nodes in the neck or under the arms – unexpressed anger and insecurity, and the person holding him or herself back from going for their goals.

Chronic Inflammation of the Tunica Albuginea (CITA) – See Peyronie's Disease

Cigarette Addiction

Since cigarette smoking results in problems with the heart and lungs, cigarette addiction represents tensions in the person's heart chakra and the area of relationships in their life, and some degree of discomfort about being loved and feeling loved. See Addiction.

Circulation Problems

In general, the blood circulatory system is associated with the heart chakra, which is the area of relationships and the person's perceptions of love – though here, it is important to consider the specific parts of the body that may have been affected. Issues with the circulation of blood in the legs, for example, could reflect tension about the circulation of love at home, or the circulation of love with the mother. Looking at the specific effects of the circulation problem can give additional insights about tensions that need to be resolved with regard to the person's perceptions of love.

Cirrhosis

Cirrhosis is scarring of the liver and poor liver function. The liver is associated with the solar plexus chakra, and therefore issues of power, control and/or freedom. Liver symptoms are associated with unreleased anger or frustration about an unhappy situation that the person feels they lack the power to change.

Claustrophobia

Claustrophobia is the fear of having no escape and being enclosed in small spaces or rooms. Claustrophobia is typically thought to have two key symptoms: fear of restriction and fear of suffocation. The fear overall points to tensions in the root chakra, the fear of restriction points to solar plexus issues (power, control, freedom) and the fear of suffocation points to heart chakra tensions (difficulty allowing in the love, not feeling loved). Together, these tensions raise questions about the area of relationships and/or perceptions of love at home. Another consideration could be crown chakra tensions with the father and/or authority and a feeling of isolation or separation, since that would also result in the sense of being in a shell and thus not feeling the love.

Clavicle

The collarbone (clavicle) is located between the ribcage (sternum) and the shoulder blade (scapula), and it connects the arm to the body. Symptoms affecting the clavicle can result in immobilization of the arm, which is associated with the throat chakra and the process of going for one's goals concerning what one wants (the will side in a right-handed person) or what will make one happy (the emotional side in a right-handed person). From the point of view that we each create our reality, rather than saying that the person cannot use their arm, we would say that the person was keeping him or herself from reaching for something. The person has a goal but has been talking to him or herself in a way that discourages them from going for that goal.

Cleft Lip, Cleft Palate

Because this is considered a birth condition caused by the baby's mouth parts not fusing or joining up during early foetal development, and because of the fact that it may affect feeding, it is important to consider the relationship between the mother and the foetus at the time the symptom began, and whether there was at that time ambivalence in the consciousness of the mother about having the child; the child might have responded to this by not feeling nourished. Another possibility could be a sense of separation from the father, resulting in a closed crown chakra and a resulting sense of isolation that could include not feeling contact with the mother.

Coccyx

The coccyx (tailbone) consists of three or more small bones fused together at the bottom of the spine. Symptoms affecting this bone reflect tensions in the root chakra, experienced as insecurity or fear, and therefore tensions in the parts of the person's consciousness concerned with security – money, home, job and their connection with their mother.

Coeliac Disease (Gluten Intolerance)

Coeliac disease is a food allergy triggered by eating foods containing gluten. It is a condition that damages the lining of the small intestine and prevents it from absorbing parts of food that are important for staying healthy. The damage is due to a reaction to eating gluten, which is found in wheat, barley, rye and sometimes oats. Coeliac disease can trigger a range of symptoms, such as:

- Diarrhoea: may be particularly unpleasant smelling; points to root chakra tensions about money, home, job or mother.
- Bloating and flatulence (passing wind): tensions in the solar plexus chakra and root chakras, reflecting possible issues of anger about root chakra parts of the person's life.
- Abdominal pain: possibly connected with the sacral chakra, but as this is still part of the elimination system it indicates root chakra tensions.
- Weight loss: the person is not allowing him or herself to be nourished.
- Feeling tired all the time (root chakra tensions): as a result of malnutrition – not getting enough nutrients from food – the person is not allowing him or herself to be nourished.
- Children not growing at the expected rate: possibly not wanting to face becoming an adult.

Generally, food allergies involving wheat and/or milk products are associated with root chakra tensions, and the person not feeling nourished by their mother. The effect of the symptom at the level of the sacral chakra reflects the person not allowing him or herself to be nourished – possibly by the love from their mother. See what was happening in the person's life at the time the symptom began, and if there are no particular tensions with the mother at that time, see other root chakra considerations – money, home, job, possibly not feeling safe at home.

Cold – See Common Cold

Cold Sores

Cold sores, sometimes called fever blisters, are groups of small blisters on the lips and around the mouth. The first symptoms of cold sores may include pain around the mouth and on the lips, a fever, a sore throat or swollen glands in the neck. Blisters and fever both indicate anger. A sore throat points to anger not expressed (What are you 'sore' about?). Swollen glands in the neck (connected with the throat chakra) point to something not expressed. All of this points to unexpressed anger, creating a symptom designed to keep others at a distance.

Colic (Baby Crying)

Infant colic is described as excessive crying in an otherwise healthy baby. The child is obviously unhappy about something but doesn't have the means to communicate what it is. There can be tensions in the solar plexus, showing anger and frustration, and this can possibly also be because of a sense of isolation (crown chakra tensions) and not feeling the contact with the parents.

Colitis

Colitis is swelling (inflammation) of the large intestine (colon). Symptoms can include: abdominal pain and bloating that either is constant or comes and goes; bloody stools; chills; constant urge to have a bowel movement.

Inflammation is associated with anger and the solar plexus chakra. The elimination system is associated with the root chakra, though part of the large intestine is located at the level of the solar plexus chakra. This condition then points to anger or frustration about the root chakra parts of the person's life – money, home, job and/or mother.

Collarbone – See Clavicle

Colon

The colon is the large intestine, and as part of the elimination system, it is associated with the root chakra and the parts of the person's consciousness related to issues of security – money, home, job. Thus, symptoms affecting the colon reflect tension in one or more of these areas. Part of the colon is located at the level of the solar plexus chakra, and since tension in the solar plexus chakra is experienced as anger, when this part of the colon is affected it can be related to anger about the root chakra parts of the person's life.

Colorectal Cancer

Any kind of cancer represents something held in and not expressed, and the part of the body affected shows what it was that was not expressed. The rectum is associated with the root chakra and therefore feeling secure or safe. Cancer of the rectum therefore points to insecurity or fear held in and not expressed, and/or the person not feeling safe at home. There can be a fear of losing something. As with any symptom, the person needs to look at what was happening in their life at the time the symptom began, which apparently was of such magnitude that the person felt they did not want to live with the situation as it was. Part of the healing must then include making a different decision, resolving the situation and having something to look forward to.

Colostomy

Colostomy is a surgical procedure that brings one end of the large intestine out through the abdominal wall, providing the person with an artificial anus. There has been tension in the root chakra, associated with the elimination system and thus tensions in the root chakra parts of the person's life – about money, home and work. When normal elimination is difficult, the person has been having issues with letting go of the root chakra tensions, letting go of the fear: 'letting go of the sh*t'. There may also be difficulty in holding their attention in the present moment.

Coma

A coma is a state of unconsciousness lasting more than six hours, in which a person: cannot be awakened; fails to respond normally to painful stimuli, light, or sound; lacks a normal sleep–wake cycle; and does not initiate voluntary actions. A person in a state of coma is described as being comatose. Although a coma patient may appear to be awake, they are unable to consciously feel, speak, hear or move; though there is a possibility that they may be aware of what is happening around them but not have the means to respond.

The person affected is unhappy about something in his or her life, has difficulty facing the situation, but has not yet made the decision to die. They are out of their body. They have let go at the level of the root chakra, which is associated with being present in their physical body and functional in the physical world. There may also be crown chakra tensions (father/authority and/or a sense of isolation) if the nervous system or the brain is affected.

Common Cold

The common cold usually causes a runny nose, nasal congestion and sneezing. The person affected may also have a sore throat, cough, headache or muscle aches.

Nasal symptoms point to root chakra tensions, and insecurity as a perceptual filter. Sore throat points to the throat chakra and unexpressed anger. Headaches point to crown chakra tensions with father/authority or a sense of separation from someone close, and muscle aches point to a perceived lack of power ('I can't...').

Concussion

Concussion (minor traumatic brain injury) is the sudden but normally short-lived loss of mental function that occurs after a blow or other injury to the head. It reflects crown chakra tension with father/authority, or a sense of separation from someone close.

Congenital Disorders – See Birth Defects

Congestion

Congestion generally means excessive crowding. Congestion may refer to issues including: congestive heart failure (heart failure due to low cardiac output); nasal congestion, throat congestion, lung congestion, chest congestion and may affect the person's relationship with air (breathing) and therefore their relationship with love, since air is the element associated with the heart chakra and perceptions of love.

The part of the body affected provides further details: nasal congestion points to root chakra tensions and difficulty letting in the love from the mother, or letting in the love at home. Throat congestion points to difficulty expressing or communicating something, and the person preventing him or herself from letting in the love. Symptoms affecting the heart, and tensions in the chest and lungs, point to heart chakra tensions with someone close to the person's heart. Generally this would be a partner, parent, sibling or child.

Conjunctivitis

Conjunctivitis (also called pink-eye or Madras eye) is inflammation of the conjunctiva (the outermost layer of the eye and the inner surface of the eyelids). The person is feeling irritated or angry about something, and prefers to avoid looking at that situation. If it is the will eye (right eye in right-handed people), it can involve something contrary to what the person wants, and if it is the other eye, the emotional eye, it is more of an emotional reaction to what they see.

Viral conjunctivitis is often associated with an infection of the upper respiratory tract, a common cold and/or a sore throat, and this points to tensions in the area of the heart chakra (relationships, perceptions of love), and the throat chakra (unexpressed anger). If it is just one eye that is affected, it should be considered as the male eye (right eye in right-handed people) or the female eye, and this could reflect tensions with a male or with a female.

Conn's Syndrome

Conn's syndrome is a disease of the adrenal glands involving excess production of a hormone called aldosterone. The primary symptom is high blood pressure, pointing to heart chakra tensions with someone close as well as root chakra tensions, since the adrenal glands are associated with the root chakra, and their activity is often triggered by fear and/or a perceived threat to survival. The symptoms may therefore point to tensions with someone at home, with sufficient intensity for the person to consider not wanting to live with the tense situation.

Constipation

Constipation is most often defined as having a bowel movement fewer than three times per week. It is associated with hard stools or difficulty passing stools. It reflects tensions in the root chakra, and therefore insecurity or fear in relation to the parts of the person's life associated with the root chakra – money, home, job – fear of letting go, fear of losing something, not feeling safe at home.

Contusion – See Bruises/Abrasions

Convulsions

A convulsion is a medical condition where body muscles contract and relax rapidly and repeatedly because of abnormal electrical activity in the brain, resulting in an uncontrolled shaking of the body. The body is out of control because of crown chakra tensions with father/authority and/or a sense of separation from someone close.

Cornea

The cornea is the transparent, dome-shaped window covering the front of the eye. Symptoms affecting the cornea can affect eyesight. The person has been reacting to tensions in their life that they find difficult to deal with, difficult to look at. If blindness is a possible logical conclusion of the symptom, the person has decided they have nothing to look forward to and feel isolated, alone. If just the male eye is affected (the right eye in right-handed people) it reflects tension with a male, and if it is the female eye, tensions with a female.

Corns

Corns, like calluses, develop from an accumulation of dead skin cells on the foot, forming thick, hardened areas. They contain a cone-shaped core with a point that can press on a nerve below, causing pain. Corns usually form on the tops, sides or tips of the toes. Corns can become inflamed due to constant friction and pressure from footwear.

Anything affecting the feet can be related to root chakra tensions (about money, home and/or job) and questions of trust. The toe(s) affected point to what the issues of trust are about. Thus, the big toe reflects the root chakra, second toe the sacral chakra, etc. In right-handed people the right foot is understood as the will foot and the left the emotional foot (this is reversed in left-handed people). Thus, a corn on the second toe of the will foot can point to issues of trust about what the person wants in the area of the sacral chakra – food or sex. A corn on the fourth toe of the emotional foot can point to issues of trust in terms of what the person feels in the area of relationships. The five toes relate to just the first five chakras, those chakras that are associated with the physical elements.

Coronary Thrombosis

A coronary thrombosis is a blood clot that goes into one of the five main coronary arteries that feed the heart itself. This would cause a heart attack or myocardial infarction by blocking the blood flow to the heart muscle. This condition is associated with tensions in the area of relationships (the heart chakra), and thus a shock to do with someone close to the person's heart – a partner, parent, sibling or child. See also Heart Attack.

Coryza

Coryza is a word describing the symptoms of a 'cold'. It describes the inflammation of the mucous membranes lining the nasal cavity that usually gives rise to the symptoms of nasal congestion and loss of smell, among other symptoms. It reflects root chakra tensions, anger (inflammation) and insecurity about money, home and/or job. See Common Cold.

Cough

The irritation might be in the chest or in the throat. When it is in the throat, it can be associated with unexpressed anger, and the person feeling irritated about something. When it is in the chest, it points more to tensions or anger with someone close to the person's heart. When someone coughs, they are pushing away air, the element associated with the heart chakra. A person's relationship with air is reflecting their relationship with love, and the person has therefore been pushing away someone's love, feeling angry with someone close to them.

Coughlan's Syndrome – See Anorgasmia

Cramps

Muscle cramps are sudden, involuntary contractions or spasms in one or more of your muscles. They reflect tensions, and the part of the body affected and the function affected reflect what the tensions are about. Thus, menstrual cramps reflect tensions about sex or about not being pregnant, or a perceived disadvantage to being a female. Leg cramps reflect root chakra tensions. See the part of the body affected for further details.

Crohn's Disease

Crohn's disease is an inflammation usually found in the last part of the small intestine and the first part of the large intestine, but it can develop anywhere in the digestive tract, from the mouth to the anus. Anything that affects the elimination system can be related to the root chakra, so this symptom can be associated with anger (inflammation) about root chakra parts of the person's life – money, home, job. If it affects the mouth, it can be seen as unexpressed anger at someone close, possibly at home (root chakra), since it would tend to discourage kissing.

Crossed Eyes

When the eyes are crossed, the person is looking inside him or herself, as if they are asking, 'What did I do?' There is a sense of guilt without knowing what the guilt is about. It is associated with having felt shocked about something at the time the symptom began, and the feeling that they must have done something wrong, even though they are not sure what it is.

Croup

Croup is a childhood condition that affects the windpipe (trachea), the airways to the lungs (the bronchi) and the voice box (larynx). It is characterized by a loud cough that resembles the barking of a seal, and difficulty breathing. It points to unexpressed anger and frustration in the child, affecting the throat and heart chakras. See Bronchitis.

Crown Chakra Tensions

The crown chakra is associated with the parts of the consciousness involving feeling connected or isolated, and also the person's relationship with authority; while of course in some families this role is assumed by the mother, the authority figure is traditionally the father. This relationship with the father is usually the model for the person's relationship with other figures of authority and, eventually, with a higher power or intelligence. Thus, a person's relationship with authority or a higher power/intelligence often mirrors their relationship with their father. A sense of separation from father or authority that closes the crown chakra results in a sense of isolation, as though the person is living in a shell.

Crown chakra tensions that could result in headaches and/or symptoms affecting the brain or nervous system include a sense of rebellion against authority or feeling the need to protect oneself from authority, or to subjugate oneself excessively to authority. A sense of separation from someone close may also result in a closed crown chakra and a sense of isolation.

Cushing's Disease, Cushing's Syndrome (Adrenal Problems)

Cushing's disease is caused by the pituitary gland (brow chakra) making too much of a hormone called ACTH, which stimulates the adrenal glands (root chakra) to make too much cortisol, a steroid stress hormone. Because the brow chakra is associated with the individualized consciousness, the person affected can consider how they feel about their gender and relate to the sex of their physical body.

Tension in the root chakra stimulating adrenal activity points to a perceived threat to survival. As always, it is important to see what was happening in the person's life at the time the symptom began, and how they may have felt threatened by or unhappy about being their gender or being in their physical body.

Cuticles

The cuticle is the strip of hardened skin at the base and sides of a fingernail or toenail. This sliver of skin acts as a protective barrier, preventing bacteria from sneaking into the nail bed and causing infection. Symptoms involving the cuticles thus can be read as affecting the fingers. See Fingers.

Cystic Fibrosis

Cystic fibrosis affects most critically the lungs, but also the pancreas, liver and intestine. The name refers to the disease's characteristic scarring (fibrosis) and cyst formation within the pancreas. Difficulty breathing is the most serious symptom. Other symptoms, including sinus infections, poor growth and infertility, affect other parts of the body.

The breathing difficulty points to tensions in the heart chakra and the person not feeling loved by someone close; having difficulty letting in that person's love. The pancreas and liver are organs that store anger, and are associated with the solar plexus chakra. Because it affects newborns it can be seen as the child's reaction to the perception of not feeling loved, and a reaction to possible ambivalence on the part of one or both of the parents about having this child at that time.

Cystitis

Cystitis is a urinary bladder inflammation, pointing to anger and insecurity about the root chakra parts of the person's life – money, home, job but most probably home. Because it can also affect sexual functioning, it can reflect insecurity concerning sexuality, or anger about a situation at home that would affect the person's attitudes toward sex.

Cystocele – See Prolapse

Cysts

A cyst is a closed sac, having a distinct membrane and division compared to the nearby tissue. It may contain air, fluids or semi-solid material. It is generically considered similar to a tumour, representing something held in and not expressed, and the part of the body affected shows what it was that had not been expressed. Thus, an ovarian cyst can point to something held in and not expressed about sex or having children, since those are the functions of the ovaries.

See the part of the body or organ affected in order to understand further details, within the context of what was happening in the person's life at the time the symptom began or was discovered or diagnosed. It is also important to consider what the effect would be if the symptom were allowed to proceed to its logical conclusion. Thus, using ovarian cysts as an example, one possibility would be that the person affected would then no longer be able to have children. Described from the point of view that we each create our reality, she has been keeping herself from having them. That would mean that she wants to have children but has been giving herself reasons not to do that at that particular time – and that would then agree with the understanding of something held in and not expressed about having children.

Dandruff

Dandruff is the shedding of dead skin cells from the scalp. While it is considered a normal condition, if it gets out of control it can reflect solar plexus issues because it controls the skin in relation to crown chakra issues – tensions with authority/father. It is likely to be background tension rather than overt conflict, but nonetheless it indicates tensions in the crown chakra.

Dark Circles Under the Eyes

Dark circles under the eyes are commonly attributed to kidney problems, anaemia, excessive smoking or drinking, allergies or sun exposure; the effect is for the person to appear tired. When the dark circles have come at a certain time in the person's life, it is interesting to ask what the person is 'tired of.' What has the person felt stressed about for too long?

Deafness

Deafness is interpreted as the person's resistance to hearing something and, as usual, it is important to consider what was happening in the person's life at the time the symptom began. If it affects the will ear (the right ear in right-handed people) it means the person is resisting hearing something contrary to what they want, and if the emotional ear is affected, it is an emotional reaction to what they are hearing. Often, it is an issue that the person does not want to hear about.

Decalcification

Decalcification is the loss of calcium from teeth and bones. When it happens with teeth they become more susceptible to cavities. When it happens with bones they become more brittle and subject to breakage. Both the teeth and the bone structure in general are associated with the root chakra and a sense of security. Loss of calcium from these areas is related to having less a sense of security – feeling insecure – and tensions in the root chakra parts of the person's life – money, home, job.

Dehydration

Dehydration is a condition that occurs when the loss of body fluids, mostly water, exceeds the amount that is taken in. Symptoms of weakness, confusion, fainting, etc. point to tensions in the root chakra parts of the person's life – money, home, job – or a perceived threat to survival. Chest pains reflect heart chakra tensions with someone close, and headaches reflect a sense of isolation or separation from someone.

Delirium

Delirium, or acute confusional state, is a syndrome that presents as severe confusion and disorientation. It reflects strong root chakra tensions of insecurity and fear and a lack of grounding. When hallucinations or delusions are present it points to altered perceptual states and a sense of isolation, reflecting crown chakra tensions with father/authority or a sense of separation from someone close.

Dementia

Dementia is the name for a group of symptoms caused by disorders that affect the brain. This points to crown chakra tensions – either tensions with authority or a sense of isolation or separation from someone. The person is living in his or her own world and may have difficulty focusing their attention on what is happening around them, pointing to root chakra tensions as well like not feeling at home and feeling insecure.

Memory loss is a common symptom of dementia. In extreme cases, the person may require constant care. Seen from the point of view that everything begins in the consciousness, the person has been making him or herself helpless, wanting to be taken care of, perhaps returning to a childhood state when that was 'normal.'

Dengue Fever

The presence of fever, rash and headache and other pains (the 'dengue triad') is particularly characteristic of dengue fever. These point to solar plexus chakra tensions including anger, and crown chakra tensions with father/authority or a sense of isolation. Other symptoms include exhaustion (root chakra tensions – insecurity, tensions at home), pain behind the eyes (difficulty looking at an unhappy situation in the person's life), severe joint and muscle pain (feeling powerless and immobilized with insecurity) and swollen lymph glands (root chakra tensions). Dengue haemorrhagic fever (fever, abdominal pain, vomiting, bleeding) is a potentially lethal complication, affecting mainly children, and reflects anger and feeling powerless and out of control.

Dependency – See Addiction

Depression

The individual feels depressed about a situation in their life about which they are unhappy but which they feel powerless to change. This points to tensions in the solar plexus chakra, associated with power, control and freedom. Often, the situation is found to be an unhappy love story, and then the person needs to stop wanting to control the situation and accept what is, moving on with their life, owning their power and their freedom and limiting their decisions to what they need to do now, rather than what someone else should do.

Dermatitis – See Eczema

Diabetes

Diabetes affects the pancreas, and a diabetic is someone who cannot have sugar. From the point of view that we each create our reality, the person has been keeping sweetness away from him or herself. If someone gets too close offering sweetness, the emotion of anger comes up to create a safe distance. Diabetes is associated with suppressed anger and comes about at a time in the person's life when they feel angry about something without the sense of freedom to express it.

Type 2 Diabetes often goes away if the person reduces their weight – the excess weight was another way to keep others at a distance.

Diaphragm

Breathing depends on the diaphragm, a sheet of muscle inside the ribcage, beneath the lungs. Symptoms affecting the diaphragm reflect solar plexus energy (anger, for example) affecting the person in the heart chakra parts of their life, and their willingness to let in the air, which represents the love from someone, since air is the element associated with the heart chakra.

Diarrhoea

Diarrhoea is the frequent passage of loose, watery, soft stools with or without abdominal bloating, pressure and cramps. It reflects tension in the root chakra, and insecurity or fear as a perceptual filter.

Digestion Difficulties

Disorders or symptoms described as digestion difficulties may involve more than the stomach, which is where digestion takes place. Stomach disorders reflect solar plexus tensions related to issues of power, control, freedom and or anger. Symptoms affecting the intestines and therefore the elimination system reflect tensions in the root chakra parts of the person's life (money, home, job) and insecurity or fear as a perceptual filter.

Diphtheria

Diphtheria usually affects the nose and throat and causes a bad sore throat, swollen glands, fever, and chills. This reflects root chakra tensions and not feeling safe at home, and throat chakra tensions and unexpressed anger. Symptoms may include hoarseness, difficulty swallowing or difficulty breathing, reflecting throat chakra tensions and heart chakra tensions – or difficulty expressing anger, possibly with someone close to the person.

Disc Herniation

A spinal disc herniation is a medical condition affecting the spine, in which a tear in the outer, fibrous ring of a disc between the vertebrae in the spine allows the soft, central portion to bulge out beyond the damaged outer rings. This can cause pressure on various nerves, causing pain. See which chakra is closest to the disc involved, and also the location of the pain. There has been tension in the affected chakra and there may be a message in the part of the body and/or the function affected by the pain. Thus, a herniated disc in the lumbar region could point to tensions at the level of the sacral chakra, about food or sex, and could represent the person immobilizing him or herself in that area of their life.

Diverticulitis, Diverticulosis

Diverticulosis happens when pouches (diverticula) form in the wall of the colon and when they get inflamed or infected it is called diverticulitis. It reflects anger (irritation) about the root chakra parts of the person's life – money, home, job.

Dizziness

Dizziness is associated with tension in the root chakra, and the person not experiencing him or herself being fully present in their physical body. This can be triggered by fear, or tension in the root chakra parts of the person's life (money, home, job) and not feeling grounded, with difficulty holding their attention in the present moment.

Dravet Syndrome/Severe Myoclonic Epilepsy of Infancy (SMEI)

Dravet syndrome, also known as severe myoclonic epilepsy of infancy (SMEI), is a form of epilepsy that begins in infancy. Development remains on track initially, with plateaus and a progressive decline typically beginning in the second year of life. Associated conditions include behavioural and developmental delays, movement and balance issues, orthopaedic conditions, delayed language and speech issues, growth and nutrition issues, sleeping difficulties and disruptions of the autonomic nervous system (which regulates things such as body temperature and sweating).

The symptoms point to crown chakra tensions and a perceived lack of contact with the child's father, and a wish to return to earlier stages of development when there was more of a sense of contact. The sense of isolation due to the closed crown chakra can also result in a sense of separation from the mother, and the root chakra symptoms.

Drug Use – See Addiction

Dry Eyes

The person with dry eyes is keeping him or herself from crying. They are unhappy about something happening in their life but do not want to show or feel the emotion.

Dry Skin

Symptoms and signs of dry skin include itching and red, cracked or flaky skin. The skin is associated with the solar plexus chakra and usually reflects how the person feels about their image, what they show the world. See the part of the body affected, and consider solar plexus issues (anger, control issues) affecting that part.

Duodenal Ulcer

A peptic ulcer is a defect in the lining of the stomach or the first part of the small intestine, an area called the duodenum. A peptic ulcer in the stomach is called a gastric ulcer. An ulcer in the duodenum is called a duodenal ulcer. Ulcers as a symptom represent anger. Common symptoms, which include bloody stools or fatigue, point to tensions or anger about the root chakra parts of the person's life – home or work. See Ulcers and Peptic Ulcer.

Duodenitis

Duodenitis is inflammation of the duodenum, the first portion of the small intestine. It reflects anger about the root chakra parts of the person's life – home, or work.

Dupuytren's Contracture

Dupuytren's contracture is a shortening and thickening of the tissue of the palm that results in clawing of the fingers. Because the hands are related to the throat chakra and the person allowing themselves to have the fulfilment of what they have asked for from the universe, this symptom can be seen as the person not allowing themselves to have this fulfilment, even if the universe has been ready to deliver it. The affected finger(s) can point to specific chakras involved with what the person has asked for. If for example, if the affected finger is the ring finger, representing the fourth chakra, it could be about fulfilment in the area of relationships; if the little finger, the area of the throat chakra, or self-expression.

Dwarfism

Dwarfism may occur if the person does not produce enough growth hormone, normally produced in the pituitary gland, associated with the brow chakra. The person may have been reluctant to come into the world, and not be happy to be here. There may have been a difficult birth. When there is physical distortion of 'normal' proportions, the person can be said to feel unattractive, unloved and isolated; in that case, crown chakra tensions would be indicated. It can be seen as a reaction on the part of the foetus to the perception of not being wanted, not feeling loved by their father.

Dysarthria – See Dysphasia

Dysentery (Amoebic or Bacillary)

Dysentery is defined as diarrhoea in which there is blood, pus and mucus, usually accompanied by abdominal pain. The two types of dysentery are symptomatically similar, and both point to tensions in the root chakra about security, survival and trust, and an emotional perceptual filter of insecurity or fear.

Dyslexia

Children and adults with dyslexia have a neurological disorder that causes their brains to process and interpret information differently, resulting in difficulty reading, writing, spelling and sometimes even speaking. It is the result of the right and left hemispheres (or the male and female parts) of the brain not communicating. It can reflect the person's reaction to tensions between their mother and father, making it difficult for the person to be open to both energies at the same time, and resulting in a closed crown chakra and a sense of isolation, as well as possible difficulties with authority.

Dysmenorrhoea

Dysmenorrhoea, or excessive menstrual pain, is associated with a perceived disadvantage to being a woman, or disappointment at not being pregnant.

Dysmorphobia

Body dysmorphic disorder, or dysmorphobia, is characterized by an unusual degree of worry or concern about a specific part of the face or body, rather than the general size or shape of the body, so in that way it is different from anorexia or bulimia. Because it is insecurity about one's appearance, it is associated with tensions in the root chakra, though the feeling of being unattractive might also be the result of a closed crown chakra (tensions with father/authority, feeling isolated) and so the person might not be feeling the love around them, not feeling loved, and might be giving themselves imaginary reasons why that is.

Dyspepsia – See Indigestion

Dysphasia/Dysarthria

Dysarthria is a disorder of speech, while dysphasia is a disorder of language. Speech itself is the process of articulation and pronunciation, involving the physical ability to form words. Language is the process in which thoughts and ideas become spoken. It involves the selection of words to be spoken, called semantics, and the formulation of appropriate sentences or phrases, called syntax.

With either symptom, the effect is for the person not to speak; from the point of view that we each create our reality, the person has been keeping him or herself from speaking, avoiding communication about something they have been unhappy about. Dysphasia is associated with the brain, and therefore points to crown chakra tensions with authority, or a feeling of isolation and separation from someone close.

Dyspnoea

Dyspnoea is shortness of breath (SOB), or 'air hunger', and is the subjective symptom of breathlessness, a feeling that one cannot breathe well enough. Because air is the element associated with the heart chakra, this condition reflects tension with someone close to the person's heart; they are not feeling the love from that individual, or have difficulties letting in the love from them because of tensions, and are feeling hungry for that love.

Dystonia

Dystonia is a neurological movement disorder characterized by spasms and sustained contractions of the muscles. These muscle movements are not under voluntary control and they result in repetitive abnormal movements of parts of the body or persistently abnormal postures. The symptoms point to a conflict between the muscles and the neurological system, and therefore between the person's sense of personal power or will and their relationship with authority; they may feel that they are obliged to follow the dictates of authority and compromise their personal power. See the muscles affected for more specific explanations. Cervical dystonia, for example, affecting the neck, points to emotions unexpressed, possibly in relation to tensions with authority.

Dysuria

Dysuria is any pain or discomfort associated with urination. It reflects root chakra tensions about money, home and work, and a sense of insecurity or fear.

Ear, Sounds in – See Tinnitus

Earache

It hurts the person to hear something or to listen to something, in terms of what was happening in the person's life when the symptom began. If it is the will ear (right ear in right-handed people) it is something contrary to what the person wants. If it is the emotional ear, it is an emotional reaction to what they have been hearing. Often, it involves not wanting to hear conflict or reacting emotionally to the conflict they hear.

Ears

In general, anything affecting the ears has something to do with the person reacting to what they have been hearing, something they do not want to hear or do not want to listen to any more. It can be about conflict or 'bad news.'

Ecchymoses

An ecchymosis is a large reddish-blue patch on the skin caused by the rupture of small blood vessels beneath the surface. It is also known as a bruise. See the part of the body affected and the chakra associated with that part of the body in order to get a sense of how the person felt 'bruised' in their consciousness in response to what was happening in their life when the symptom occurred. See also Bruises/Abrasions.

Ectopic Pregnancy

An ectopic pregnancy is a pregnancy that occurs outside the womb (uterus). It is a life-threatening condition for the mother, and the baby (foetus) cannot survive. This can be related to ambivalence in the consciousness of the mother about being pregnant and bringing a child into her present circumstances. There may be questions about the stability of the family, or questions of freedom or how life might be adversely affected by the birth of the child.

Eczema or Dermatitis

Eczema, also called dermatitis, is a term for several different types of skin swelling. Typically, eczema shows itself as patches of chronically itchy, dry, thickened skin, usually on the hands, neck, face and legs. The part of the body affected and the chakra associated with that part point to specific sensitivities. The hands being affected can reflect nervousness or irritation about accepting the fulfilment of their goals. The neck being affected reflects unexpressed irritation. When the face is affected, it reflects a sense of shame or guilt since the person may feel they need to hide their face. If it is on the legs, it reflects nervous insecurity or lack of trust.

People with atopic dermatitis often also have asthma or seasonal allergies, and all this together points to heart chakra sensitivities and tensions in the person's perceptions of love or tensions with someone close. There may be a family history of allergic conditions such as asthma, hay fever or eczema. Hay fever and asthma point to sensitivities about allowing in the love, often the love from the mother, reflecting tensions there.

Elbows

Because the elbows are associated with the throat chakra, and the arms with setting goals, symptoms affecting the elbows point to the person talking him or herself out of going for their goals. Typically at the time the symptom began there were specific goals, but the person convinced him or herself not to go for them.

Embolism

As a blood clot moves through the body's blood vessels, it may come to a passage it does not fit through and can lodge there, backing up blood behind it. The cells that normally get their blood supply via this passage can then be starved of oxygen and die. This condition is called an embolism. The blood circulatory system is related to the heart chakra and therefore to the person's perceptions of love. The part of the body affected points to the specific tension in the consciousness of the person affected. Thus, if the brain is affected, it points to crown chakra tensions and a sense of separation from someone close. If the lungs are affected it points to tensions with someone close to the person's heart – partner, parent, sibling or child. If the person's eyes are affected, the right (male) or left (female) eye, depending on whether the person was right- or left-handed, would reflect them not seeing the male or the female in their life; a sense of separation from a male or female at the time the symptom began.

Emphysema

In people with emphysema, the tissues necessary to support the physical shape and function of the lungs are destroyed. Breathing is affected, and this points to tensions in the heart chakra, associated with the element of air. A person's relationship with air mirrors their relationship with love – difficulty allowing it in (difficulty feeling loved), or difficulty letting it out (difficulty expressing love). Thus, there have been tensions with someone close to the person.

Encephalitis

Encephalitis is irritation and swelling (inflammation) of the brain, pointing to tensions in the crown chakra and thus tensions with father/authority and/or a sense of isolation and not feeling the love around them.

End Plate Sclerosis

End plate sclerosis is a medical term that refers to an increased thickening or density at the top and bottom of a vertebra. It is considered a sign of disc degeneration, and commonly occurs in the early stages of osteoarthritis. See which part of the spine is affected, and which chakra is associated with that part, as well as which function might be affected by the symptom. Because the spine in general is associated with the root chakra, it reflects insecurity in the affected area. Thus, if the condition is located at the level of the sacral chakra it could reflect insecurity about food, sex or having children. If the effect is immobilization, the person has been immobilizing him or herself in that area because of insecurity.

Endocarditis

Endocarditis is an inflammation of the inner layer of the heart, the endocardium. It usually involves the heart valves (native or prosthetic valves). It reflects tensions with someone close, and the severity of the symptom reflects the degree of unhappiness about the situation.

Endometriosis

Endometriosis is a female health disorder that occurs when cells from the lining of the womb (uterus) grow in other areas of the body. This can lead to pain, irregular bleeding and problems getting pregnant. These other cells can grow on the ovaries, bowel, rectum, bladder and the lining of the pelvic area. These symptoms point to tensions in the root and sacral chakras, insecurities about getting pregnant or having a child, and possible tensions at home.

Enteric Fever

Typhoid fever, also known as enteric fever, is a potentially fatal illness. The classic presentation includes fever, malaise, diffuse abdominal pain and constipation. Symptoms may include intestinal haemorrhage, bowel perforation and death within one month of onset. It reflects solar plexus tensions of anger and strong root chakra symptoms: not feeling safe at home.

Enterobiasis – See Pinworms

Enuresis – See Bed-Wetting

Epicondylalgia/Epicondylitis (Tennis Elbow)

Lateral epicondylalgia or lateral epicondylitis, known colloquially as tennis elbow, shooter's elbow and archer's elbow or simply lateral elbow pain, is a condition where the outer part of the elbow becomes sore and tender. The arms are associated with the throat chakra and represent the person's attitudes about going for their goals. The person has been talking him or herself out of going for a specific goal. The symptom is associated with overexertion, and this can point to a possible conflict of goals between the apparent outer cause (the specific activity – tennis, for example) and another part of the person's life that might be in conflict with the activity, since the effect of the symptom can be to discontinue the activity. From the point of view that we create our reality, the person has been keeping him/herself from playing tennis (or golf, or archery). In any event they are trying too hard with something that should be a passion, an expression of something they love to do and should be doing for its own sake, not with tensions.

Epidemics

From the point of view that everything begins in the consciousness, epidemics of a particular symptom reflect tensions in the group consciousness that the individual has accepted. See the symptom involved to understand the group consciousness value that the individual has accepted.

Epilepsy

Epilepsy is a brain disorder in which a person has repeated seizures (convulsions) over time. The brain is associated with the crown chakra and the relationship with father/authority. The person goes out of their body, letting go at the level of the root chakra. The symptom is often triggered by fear. There is apparent separation between the crown and root chakras, which reflects the person's relationship with their mother. The person experiences excessive activity in their crown chakra (father) in relation to a separation from the root chakra (mother). The person may have reacted to what was happening between their father and their mother at that time, and possibly to not feeling safe at home.

Epiphysis

Slipped capital femoral epiphysis (SCFE) is an unusual disorder of the adolescent hip. The ball at the upper end of the femur (thigh bone) slips off in a backward direction. Most often, this develops during periods of accelerated growth, shortly after the onset of puberty. It occurs two to three times more often in males than females. A large number of patients are overweight for their height. All of this points to root chakra tensions and insecurity related to adolescence and puberty, and the person's attitudes toward their emerging sexuality.

Epstein–Barr Virus

EBV is the cause of infectious mononucleosis (also termed 'mono'), an illness associated with fever, sore throat, swollen lymph nodes in the neck and sometimes an enlarged spleen, all of which points to tensions in the solar plexus and throat chakras. It is associated with unexpressed anger, or insecurity about expressing anger when the lymph nodes in the neck have been affected.

Erectile Dysfunction – See Impotence

Excrescence

An excrescence is an outgrowth or enlargement, especially an abnormal one, disfiguring or unwanted, such as warty excrescences in the colon. Any growth can be seen as representing something held in and not expressed, with the part of the body affected showing what it was that was not expressed. If a function is affected, such as with a growth in the colon, see which chakra is affected; in this case, for example, it would affect the elimination system and therefore would reflect tensions in the root chakra parts of the person's life – money, home, job.

Exotropia – See Crossed Eyes

Eyelids

When the eyelids are affected, the symptom can result in the eyelid closing and the person thus not seeing through that eye. The right eye in right-handed people is considered the will eye or the male eye and vision difficulties with this eye can be associated with the person keeping him or herself from seeing clearly what they want, or not seeing the male in their life – feeling separated from a man or men in general – at the time the symptom began. The other eye is the emotional eye or the female eye, and difficulties with this eye are related to the person avoiding seeing clearly what they feel, or not seeing the female in their life. If both eyelids are affected, it can look like the person is crying – unhappy about a situation in their life.

Eyes, General

The eyes are associated with the solar plexus chakra, and therefore with ease of being. Someone with impaired eyesight is therefore not easy in their way of being, and the different kinds of impaired eyesight give details about the stressed way of being that the person has adopted in response to conditions in their life at the time the vision was affected. See the specific vision disorders in this listing for an explanation of the personality profile associated with that particular disorder.

The right eye in right-handed people is considered the will eye or the male eye and vision difficulties with this eye can be associated with the person keeping him or herself from seeing clearly what they want, or not seeing the male in their life; there were tensions involving a male at the time the symptom began. The other eye is the emotional eye or the female eye, and difficulties with this eye can be related to the person avoiding seeing clearly what they feel, or tensions involving a female, not seeing the female in their life.

When the two eyes are not working together, it is seen as the male and the female not communicating, and this can be related to the person's reaction to a non-harmonious polarity between his or her parents.

Eyesight, General

Eyesight can be related to the solar plexus chakra and perceptions of power, control and freedom, as well as ease of being for the person, not feeling threatened by what they see. Impaired eyesight reflects tension in the consciousness and a perception of a threatening world in which it is not safe to be who you really are, as if being yourself and living your truth carries with it an implied threat. See the particular eyesight symptom for further details.

Face

The face in general is associated with what the person shows the world, and reflects how they feel they appear to others, their self-definition and therefore the solar plexus chakra. Specific parts of the face, though, relate to different chakras, and symptoms affecting those parts relate to tensions in those chakras. The nose relates to the root chakra, the tongue to the second and fifth chakras (food and communication), lips to the throat chakra, ears to the throat chakra. Cheeks would relate to the skin and the solar plexus chakra, and when these are affected by acne, for example, the person is making him or herself unattractive – not wanting to risk being attractive – because of a perceived threat to their way of being when they are sexual or in a relationship.

Facial Nerves, Facial Palsy

The facial nerves control the muscles of the face, and when those are affected, as with Bell's palsy, a form of facial paralysis occurs through a dysfunction of the facial nerve that results in the inability to control facial muscles on the affected side. The person has felt deeply insulted ('slapped in the face') as a response to an event in their life. See Bell's Palsy.

Fainting/Blackouts

When someone faints, they let go at the level of the root chakra and they go out of their body. This can be triggered by fear or worry about something. It also can reflect weaknesses or tensions in the root chakra parts of the person's life (money, home, job, mother) as a predisposing factor.

Fallen Arches – See Flat Feet

Fallopian Tubes

The Fallopian tubes are the small ducts that link a woman's ovaries to her uterus and are part of the reproductive system. Symptoms reflect ambivalent feelings about having children. On the will side (the right side in people born right-handed) the symptom points to a conflict between her will and what her body is asking for, and on the emotional side, an emotional reaction to what her body is asking for as a possible violation of her values.

Far-sightedness

People who are far-sighted see what is further away from them more easily than what is close to them. Far-sighted people are more focused on what is outside themselves and less on what is inside. Energy – the direction of attention – is expanding and moving outward, holding away or moving against what is outside. Things must be held at a distance to be seen clearly and comfortably. Giving can seem more important than receiving, as though what others want or feel is more important than the individual's own wants or feelings, and there is an excessive orientation toward others and away from Self. 'You' is considered more important than 'I', and 'we' does not seem to include 'I' as an equal consideration.

A far-sighted person may be interested in other people's lives, avoiding looking at their own. Their image (how they appear to others) may be overemphasized and identified with, gaining more importance to them than their essence, the person behind the image – who they really are. Anger or guilt are perceptual filters, though any sense of anger may be suppressed, so as not to offend others. The focus of thinking is in the past, often with anger and self-justification, or else a sense of not having done 'the right thing.' This preoccupation with the past keeps the individual from being totally present. The degree to which this is true is a matter of individual balance, and the degree of far-sightedness experienced by the individual.

There is tension in the solar plexus chakra and the throat chakra.

Farting – See Flatulence

Fat

Fat is not in itself a problem unless it reaches a degree of affecting the person's health and/or mobility. If it affects the person's mobility, it could be said that they have been immobilizing themselves. If it affects the person's health because of possible heart problems, it could reflect tensions in the area of relationships with people close to their heart. If the person feels unattractive, they have been making themselves unattractive because of sensitivities in the area of the heart chakra or sacral chakra, sensitivities about love or sex and not wanting to deal with the risks of being attractive.

Fatigue

Fatigue in general or experiencing low levels of energy reflects root chakra tensions about money, home and/or job, or other root chakra tensions (survival, trust). The person can ask him or herself what they are 'tired of.'

Feet

The feet are associated with the root chakra. The right foot in right-handed people is considered to be the will foot or the male foot, and the other foot is the emotional foot or the female foot. Symptoms affecting just one foot can then be said to reflect lack of trust in a man, for the male foot, or lack of trust in a female, for the female foot, or else a lack of trust in the will (for the will foot), or in the foundations of the emotional being (for the emotional foot). Lack of trust in the will implies that the person has made a decision but has not acted on it, not insisted, not 'put their foot down', because of insecurity; and lack of trust in the area of emotions can imply a sense of emotional insecurity or dependency, not standing on one's own two feet with regard to one's emotions.

The possible logical conclusion of the symptom if it were allowed to advance needs to be examined as well. If the person would not be able to walk, for example, it could be said that they have been keeping themselves from walking away from a situation they have been unhappy with, giving themselves reasons to stay in the unhappy situation.

Felon/Whitlow

An infection inside the tip of the finger can form an enclosed pocket of pus (or abscess) that is very painful as it expands. A felon is a fingertip abscess deep in the palm side of the finger. An abscess reflects anger, possibly preventing the person achieving a particular goal. See Fingers for details of what the anger is about.

Fever

Fever implies anger. The element associated with the solar plexus chakra is fire. The person is angry about something happening in their life.

Fever Blisters – See Cold Sores

Fibroid Tumours

Fibroids are considered symptomatically similar to tumours, in that they represent something held in and not expressed, and the part of the body affected shows what it was that was not being expressed. When the fibroids affect the uterus, this can reflect tension or ambivalence about having children, though the physical location also points to tensions in the root chakra, and therefore issues of trust with a man. See Cysts.

Fibromyalgia/Painful Muscles

Fibromyalgia is associated with muscular and joint pain, sensitivity to pressure in particular points and fatigue. This points to solar plexus issues involving the person not owning their power, and also root chakra tensions. The person has been immobilizing him or herself through insecurity. The elimination system may be affected, again pointing to root chakra tensions about money, home, job or tensions with their mother. The location of the sensitive points on the body can be the throat and chest and arms, pointing to tension in the throat and heart chakras, reflecting difficulty communicating with someone close and uncertainty about setting future goals. If there is fatigue (root chakra) it could reflect tensions with someone close to their heart at home.

Fingernails – See Nails

Fingers

Each of the fingers relates to a chakra, with the thumb representing the root chakra, index finger representing the sacral chakra, etc. Only the first five chakras are represented in this way. The right hand in a right-handed person is the will hand, and the left is the emotional hand. The symptoms are read from the throat chakra, which controls the arms and hands. Thus, the thumb on the will hand represents something about expressing what one wants in relation to the root chakra parts of their life – money, home, job. The index finger on the will hand represents something about expressing what the person wants in relation to food or sex. The middle finger on the will hand represents something about the person expressing what they want concerning power, control or freedom. The ring finger on the will hand represents something about the person expressing what they want in terms of the heart chakra and the area of relationships, and the little finger on the will hand represents something about the person expressing what they want in terms of how they express themselves (this could be about creative expression, for example).

On the emotional hand, the thumb would represent expressing feelings about root chakra issues, the index finger feelings about food or sex, the middle finger feelings about power, control and freedom, the ring finger feelings about the area of relationships; and the little finger would represent expressing feelings about how the person expresses themselves.

Fishskin Disease

Ichthyosis vulgaris or fishskin disease is a skin disorder in which dead skin cells accumulate in thick, dry scales on the skin's surface. The scales are usually not detected at birth but, as the child grows older, dry scaling will appear, being most marked on the extremities. See at what age the scaling appeared, and tensions about what was happening in the child's family life at that time and/or their sense of connection with their parents.

The symptom may be associated with a deficiency of the sweat glands and, less frequently, with irregularities in the growth of hair, teeth and nails, pointing to tensions in the root and crown chakras, and thus tensions with the parents. People afflicted with mild cases have symptoms that include scaly patches on the shins, fine white scales on the forearms and upper arms and rough palms, pointing to solar plexus energy affecting the root chakra and throat chakras, and thus insecurity and uncertainty about one's future.

Fissure

An anal fissure is a tear in the lining of the lower rectum (anus) that causes pain during bowel movements and reflects root chakra tensions about money, home and/or job.

Fistula

A fistula is an abnormal connection or passageway between organs or vessels that normally do not connect. It can affect various organs throughout the body, and the organ affected points to the specific tension in the person's consciousness related to the symptom.

For example, an anal fistula could cause pain and bleeding when one goes to the toilet, and would point to root chakra tensions and insecurities about money, home and/or job.

Flat Feet

A person with flat feet has low arches or no arches at all. The arch is the inside part of the foot that is usually raised off the ground when standing normally. This condition reflects root chakra tensions and the person not feeling 'supported.'

Flatulence

Flatulence or farting is caused by intestinal gas, and is a normal condition. When it is excessive, it can be related to excessive activity in the solar plexus chakra, reflecting control issues and/or anger, and possible root chakra tensions (money, home, job, mother).

Flu – See Influenza

Food Poisoning

Possible symptoms of food poisoning include diarrhoea (may be bloody), pointing to root chakra tensions, insecurity and not feeling safe at home; fever and chills, which point to anger and solar plexus tensions; headache, pointing to crown chakra issues with father/authority or a sense of isolation; nausea and vomiting, pointing to feeling out of control and weakness, indicating tensions in the solar plexus and root chakras, feeling powerless to change an unhappy situation.

Foot Problems – See Feet

Forehead

Because the brow chakra is located at the level of the forehead, tensions there can be related to the person inside the body not feeling that they are seen, because people relate to their body or to their role rather than to them as a person.

It can also be due to tensions in the area of spirituality and religion, or the person not feeling comfortable with the functions at this level of consciousness, which can include ESP and spirit-to-spirit communication.

Forgetfulness

Forgetfulness points to root chakra tensions about money, home or job, and a sense of not being fully present, not being grounded.

Fractures

A fracture is a broken bone, and to understand the inner cause of the symptom, it is necessary to see the location of the broken bone, and which chakra is associated with that part of the body, as well as which function is affected. How does the person experience the effects of the fracture? How do they feel limited? Describing it from the point of view that the person created it gives insight into the inner cause.

Friedrich's Ataxia

Friedrich's ataxia symptoms are caused by the wearing away of structures in areas of the brain and spinal cord that control coordination, muscle movement and some sensory functions. This points to crown chakra tensions with father/authority and/or a sense of separation from someone close. Symptoms generally begin in childhood before puberty, and may include abnormal speech, changes in vision, decrease in ability to feel vibrations in lower limbs, foot problems, such as hammer toe and high arches, hearing loss, loss of coordination and balance, which leads to frequent falls, muscle weakness (feeling powerless), unsteady gait and uncoordinated movements (ataxia) that gets worse with time and muscle problems that lead to changes in the spine, which may result in scoliosis.

All of this points to the sense of isolation as the result of tensions with authority or separation from someone close, and various effects of that in the root chakra, creating a sense of insecurity and helplessness. Heart disease usually develops as the result of the person not feeling the love around them, and may lead to heart failure, from which death may result. Diabetes may develop in later stages of the disease, reflecting anger at someone and not allowing others to get close; this can be seen as another effect of the isolation of the crown chakra tension.

Frigidity

Frigidity, in psychology, is the inability of a woman to attain orgasm during sexual intercourse. In popular, non-medical usage the word has been used traditionally to describe issues from general coldness of manner or lack of interest in physical affection to aversion to sexual intercourse. When it is about an aversion to sex, it is clearly about the sacral chakra, which governs the gonads and the messages from the physical body to the person inside the body.

When it is about difficulty reaching orgasm, it could also reflect tension in the root chakra, and the person having difficulty letting go into the orgasm.

When it is about general coldness of manner or lack of interest in physical affection it can point to tensions in the heart chakra and perceptions of love, since the physical sense associated with the heart chakra is the sense of touch – though there might also be crown chakra issues resulting in the person experiencing a sense of isolation, as if they are in a shell, not feeling the contact with others outside the shell; this can be the result of a sense of separation from their father. See also Hypogyneismus.

Fungus, Fungal Infections

A fungus eats, and a fungal infection can be seen as something 'eating away' at the person, bothering them in the background of their consciousness. The part of the body affected points to what it is. For example, athlete's foot is a fungal infection, and indicates some background tension eating away at the person's sense of security (root chakra). A vaginal yeast infection can similarly point to root chakra issues, but since it also affects the person's sexual activity, it can be seen as something bothering the person in the background of their attitudes about sex.

Furuncles – See Boils

G6PD Deficiency

Considered a hereditary condition, glucose-6-phosphate dehydrogenase (G6PD) deficiency is where red blood cells break down when the body is exposed to certain drugs or the stress of infection. This points to the person not allowing him or herself to be nourished by the love around them, possibly because of crown chakra issues like tension with father/authority, a sense of separation from their father or a sense of isolation, leaving them feeling as though they are in a shell and therefore not feeling the love around them.

Gall-Bladder Calculosis (Gallstones)

The gall bladder is associated with the solar plexus chakra and is one of the organs associated with anger, and this symptom represents the person's difficulty with expressing anger.

Ganglioglioma – See Brain Tumour

Ganglion Cyst

A ganglion cyst is a benign soft tissue tumour that may occur in any joint, but most often occurs on or around the joints and tendons in the hands or feet. Any cyst represents something held in and not expressed. Affecting the hands, it represents the person talking to him or herself in a way that gives them reasons to avoid having something they have asked for from the universe. Affecting the feet, it can represent issues of mistrust with a male (if it is the male foot, the right foot in right-handed people) or with a female (affecting the female foot), or the person not insisting on trusting their will, not 'putting their foot down' (will foot, right foot in right-handed persons), or emotional insecurity (affecting the emotional foot).

Gangrene

Gangrene is the death of tissue in a part of the body. It happens when a body part loses its blood supply. This may happen through injury, an infection or other causes. To understand the inner cause of the symptom, we need to see what part of the body is affected; this will indicate which is the chakra and function associated with that part, and what it is that is 'dying' in their consciousness.

Gas Pains

To understand the inner cause of gas pains, see where in the body the person experiences the pain, and which chakra is closest to that part.

Because the gas is caused by digestive activity, it points to solar plexus energy or tension (anger, for example) affecting that person in that part of their consciousness. If there is severe stomach pain, it is tension about power or control, or anger issues. On the right side of the body, the pain is understood as an inner conflict on the will side of the solar plexus (conflict of will within the context of power, control, freedom – the person fighting within themselves about what they want) or sacral chakra (deciding what the body should have rather than listening to the body). When the pain is on the left side, it is an emotional conflict in these areas. If it is on the upper left, it can be mistaken for a heart problem, or an emotional conflict in the area of relationships.

Gastritis

Gastritis occurs when the lining of the stomach becomes inflamed or swollen. Inflammation indicates anger. Symptoms affecting the stomach, associated with the solar plexus chakra, point to tensions involving control issues.

Gastroenteritis

Gastroenteritis is a condition that causes irritation and inflammation of the stomach and intestines. Symptoms include vomiting and diarrhoea, and reflect tensions in the solar plexus and root chakras, and therefore anger and insecurity about the root chakra parts of the person's life – money, home and work.

Gastrointestinal Symptoms

Gastrointestinal (GI) disturbances commonly include symptoms of stomach pain, heartburn, diarrhoea, constipation, nausea and vomiting. See the individual symptoms for details about the inner cause.

Generalized Anxiety Disorder (GAD)

Generalized anxiety disorder or GAD is characterized by excessive, exaggerated anxiety and worry about everyday life events when there are no obvious reasons for worrying. People with symptoms of GAD tend to always expect disaster and can't stop worrying about health, money, family, work or school. The symptom points to tension in the root chakra, related to the parts of the person's consciousness concerned with security, survival, trust and the parts of the person's life concerned with security – money, home and job. The root chakra also reflects the person's sense of connection with their mother, thus it becomes interesting to see when the GAD began, and what was happening in the person's life in these areas at the time.

Genetic Disorders

As with any symptoms, those considered to be genetic or hereditary disorders are associated with specific tensions in the person's consciousness related to what was happening in their life at the time the symptom was detected.

Children learn from observing their parents. When the conditions in a parent's consciousness predispose them to a particular condition, and the child imitates or copies that way of being, they can then be predisposed to the same symptom. When the child changes their way of being, the conditions for the symptom no longer exist, and can be released, according to whatever the person allows themselves to believe is possible; and there are examples of 'genetic' symptoms such as diabetes and colour blindness that have been released when there have been strong changes in the person's consciousness.

The genetic structure is a molecular chain with open links onto which one of several different ions can attach, and this represents the code with which information is written there. Thus, the genetic structure is a record of past experiences, which can represent a predisposition to a particular condition; this is not inviolable, though, and since we continue to experience, we continue to write information onto the genetic structure. Though the genetic structure may be statistically correlated with the symptom, it does not explain why the symptom appeared at a particular time in the person's life. Thus, it is still important to see what was happening in the person's life at the time the symptom began or was discovered, and recognize the symptom as reflecting tension in the person's consciousness in response to those conditions at that time.

Genital Herpes – See Herpes

Genital Warts – See Human Papillomavirus (HPV)

Genitals

The genitals (testicles in men, ovaries in women) are associated with the sacral chakra and involved with sex and having children.

Symptoms involving the gonads (genitals), then, reflect tensions in the person's consciousness in these specific areas in response to what was happening in the person's life at the time the symptom began.

German Measles – See Rubella

Gigantism – See Acromegaly

Gingivitis

Gum disease, also known as gingivitis or periodontal disease, is a condition in which the gums become swollen, sore or infected. Symptoms affecting the gums and/or teeth are related to root chakra tensions about money, home and work, and possibly mother, and gingivitis points to anger (feeling 'sore') about the root chakra parts of the person's life at the time the symptom began.

Glandular Fever (Infectious Mononucleosis)

Infectious mononucleosis (also termed 'mono') is an illness associated with fever, sore throat, swollen lymph nodes in the neck and sometimes an enlarged spleen, pointing to tensions in the solar plexus and throat chakras. It reflects unexpressed anger as well as a sense of isolation, since it is considered very contagious, and this can also reflect crown chakra tensions with father/authority. See Mononucleosis.

Glaucoma

Glaucoma is pressure in the eye that can build up to the point where it damages the optic nerve. The person has a pressured way of seeing the world and could benefit from relaxation techniques. There is tension in the solar plexus chakra, which is associated with eyesight. Because it can result in blindness, which also results in a sense of isolation, or separation from someone, it can reflect crown chakra tensions and the person feeling pressured and that they must deal with their life issues alone.

Gluten Intolerance

Gluten intolerance is associated with tensions in the root chakra and in the person's sense of not feeling nourished by their mother. See Coeliac Disease.

Goitre (Thyroid)

Goitre is an enlargement of the thyroid gland, and points to tension in the throat chakra, which is related to expression. There is something the person has difficulty expressing. If it affects swallowing, there is difficulty in 'swallowing' or accepting some unhappy condition in the person's life at the time the symptom began. If it results in a cough, it reflects unexpressed anger. If there is accompanying hyperthyroidism (overactive thyroid) or hypothyroidism (underactive thyroid), the person has been giving him or herself reasons not to express naturally and easily who they really are.

Gonorrhoea

Gonorrhoea is a sexually transmitted disease, and its symptoms include difficulty when urinating, sensitivity in the affected area (sexual organs) and, often, a sore throat. This points to tension not only in the sacral chakra, related to sex, but also in the root chakra (insecurity or fear) and unexpressed anger (throat chakra). It also indicates that the person is conflicted in their attitude toward their sexuality.

Gout

Gout is a kind of arthritis that occurs when uric acid builds up in the blood and causes joint inflammation. Acute gout is a painful condition that typically affects one or a few joints. The big toe, knee or ankle joints are most often affected. All of this points to tension in the root chakra, and thus the parts of the person's consciousness concerned with money, home and job. See which specific part is affected, and whether it is on the will side or emotional side, for further details about the person's reaction to what was happening in their life when the symptom began.

Graves' Disease

Graves' disease is described as an autoimmune disease where the thyroid is overactive. The thyroid gland is associated with the throat chakra, which is about expressing oneself. When this gland is overactive, the person is over-expressing. There is a way in which they do not feel safe to show who they really are, and they are projecting an overactive persona that is not their natural one. See what was happening in this person's life when the symptom began, and what the conditions were that they responded to by deciding that it was not safe to show who they really are, nor to express their truth.

Groin

The groin is a term for the crease or hollow at the junction of the inner part of each thigh with the trunk, together with the adjacent region and often including the external genitalia. Symptoms affecting this area reflect tensions in the root chakra parts of the person's life (money, home, job), as well as possible tensions about sex or having children, if the symptoms discourage sexual activity.

Growths

Growths are considered generically and symptomatically like tumours, in that they represent something held in and not expressed, with the part of the body affected reflecting what it is that has been held in and not expressed, in terms of which chakra and/or function is associated with that part. See the part affected for further details.

Guillain–Barré Syndrome

Guillain–Barré syndrome is a condition of the peripheral nervous system, the network of nerves that lies outside the central nervous system including the motor nerves, which the brain uses to control the muscles. In this syndrome, the immune system (the body's natural defence against infection and illness) attacks these nerves, causing them to become inflamed and stop working. The nervous system points to crown chakra tensions, and the muscles are related to the solar plexus chakra and perceptions of power. Thus, the symptoms point to a perceived lack of power when facing authority. Possible involvement of the immune system, related to the heart chakra, points to tensions with an authority close to the person's heart, usually the father.

The symptoms of Guillain–Barré syndrome usually develop one to three weeks after a minor infection, such as a cold, sore throat or gastroenteritis (an infection of the stomach and bowel), and these symptoms point to anger. Symptoms often start in the feet and hands before spreading to the arms and then the legs, pointing to root chakra tensions and difficulty setting goals. Initially, the person may have pain, tingling and numbness, progressive muscle weakness, coordination problems and unsteadiness (difficulty walking unaided), again reflecting root chakra tensions.

The symptoms reflect tensions with an authority at home that is negatively affecting the person's sense of power to decide their future.

Gums

Symptoms affecting the gums are related to weakness in the root chakra, and therefore tension in the parts of the person's consciousness concerned with what represents security in their life, money, home and work. The person does not have strong roots or a great sense of security.

Haematemesis

Haematemesis is the vomiting of blood, which may either be obviously red or have an appearance similar to coffee grounds. Haematemesis indicates that the bleeding is from the upper gastrointestinal tract, usually from the oesophagus, stomach or proximal duodenum. This reflects solar plexus tensions, strong anger about conditions that exist in the person's life that they find difficult to accept and feel they cannot control, possibly in the area of relationships.

Haematoma

A haematoma is a collection of blood, usually clotted, outside of a blood vessel, that may occur because of an injury to the wall of a blood vessel, allowing blood to leak out into tissues where it does not belong. Blood that escapes from the bloodstream is very irritating and may cause symptoms of inflammation including pain, swelling and redness. Symptoms of a haematoma depend upon its location, its size and whether it causes associated swelling. See the part of the body or the function affected to understand how the person felt 'bruised', and the decisions they made as the result of having felt 'bruised' or 'irritated' by what happened in their life when the symptom began. See also Subdural Haematoma.

Haematuria

Haematuria is blood in the urine, which can be from anywhere along the urinary elimination system: the kidneys, ureters (the tubes that transport urine from the kidneys to the bladder), bladder or urethra. It all points to tensions in the root chakra parts of the person's life (money, home, job) and, if the kidneys are the organs affected, a sense of helplessness with the feeling that the person can not do anything about the situation they have been unhappy about.

Haemophilia

Haemophilia is a bleeding disorder in which the blood doesn't clot normally, resulting in abnormal bleeding. Because it affects the blood it is associated with the heart chakra. The person affected feels easily hurt by conflicts with people close to their heart.

Haemoptysis

Haemoptysis is the spitting of blood that originated in the lungs or bronchial tubes. It points to extreme anger in the area of relationships (heart chakra) with people close to the person's heart – typically a partner, parent, sibling or child.

Haemorrhage

To haemorrhage is to undergo heavy or uncontrollable bleeding. The blood circulatory system is related to the heart chakra, and therefore to the person's perceptions of love. Excessive bleeding can be life-threatening, therefore something the person feels bad enough about to consider dying. The part of the body affected reflects the difficult situation in the person's life at the time the symptom began, in which the person may have felt a lack of love. Thus, haemorrhaging from the nose, associated with the root chakra, represents the person not feeling safe at home. Menstrual haemorrhaging reflects tensions about the area of having children. For haemorrhaging from a wound, see the part of the body affected for further details.

Haemorrhoids

Haemorrhoids are painful, swollen veins in the lower portion of the rectum or anus. They point to tensions in the root chakra, and thus about the parts of the person's life related to security issues – worry about money, home, work. There is fear of losing something.

Hair (Excessive, Baldness, etc.)

The hair in general is associated with the crown chakra and, when there is hair loss, it points to crown chakra tensions with father/authority or a sense of separation or isolation. Excessive hair or male-pattern baldness in women also reflects crown chakra tension, since it creates a sense of isolation, though it can also point to sacral chakra tensions concerning sexuality, or heart chakra tensions about being in a relationship, and possible dissatisfaction with the female role or being in a female body.

Halitosis – See Bad Breath

Hallucinations

A hallucination is defined as a perception occurring without any identifiable external stimulus and is generally considered an abnormality in perception. By this definition, in a society in which all non-ordinary experiences are given a pathological label, all extrasensory perceptions (ESP) and many valid spiritual experiences are considered hallucinations, as are religious experiences of talking with God or angels, which have in fact been the basis of forming some religions. ESP and spirit-to-spirit communication are related to the brow chakra and, while non-ordinary, may not be 'abnormalities' unless they are labelled as such, and then the problem may be the pejorative label and the person feeling that there is something wrong with them, until they can understand their perceptions within a different context.

If the non-ordinary perceptions result in difficulty functioning within society, and a sense of isolation, or if there is brain damage associated with the hallucinations, it points to crown chakra tensions with father/authority or a sense of separation from someone close, and the person closed in their own world.

Hands, General

The hands in general are associated with the throat chakra, and with the person's ability or willingness to receive or to let him or herself have the delivery of something they have asked for. The person has asked for a goal, or prayed for something, the delivery is possible and they have been giving themselves reasons not to allow themselves to have the fulfilment of that goal, or to believe they can not have the fulfilment of that goal.

Hansen's Disease – See Leprosy

Harelip – See Cleft Lip, Cleft Palate

Hay Fever

Hay fever (allergic rhinitis) involves irritation and inflammation of the mucous membrane inside the nose. Common symptoms are a stuffy nose, runny nose and post-nasal drip. Hay fever is usually triggered on the physical level by airborne allergens such as pollen.

Because it is the nose that has been affected, the symptom is related to the root chakra and specifically tension in the relationship with the mother. Because it involves taking in air through the nose, and that air is the element associated with the heart chakra and one's perceptions of love, it can be related to difficulty letting in the love from the mother.

There may be additional symptoms, such as sneezing and nasal itching, coughing – the person is pushing away the air and therefore the love, they may be angry at someone close to them. When the person has headaches it indicates tensions in the crown chakra, which can be tensions with their father and/or authority, or because of a sense of separation or isolation.

Fatigue and cognitive impairment, where the person does not think clearly, are associated with root chakra tensions; the person has no roots, no sense of security. The eyes may also be affected, being watery, reddened or itchy and with puffiness around them; the person looks like they are crying, signifying unhappiness about something and the person finding it difficult to look at something happening in their life.

Head, General

When we are discussing symptoms related to the head, we mean the part of the head above the face. In general, the head is associated with the crown chakra, and therefore with the parts of the person's consciousness concerned with father/authority and the sense of separation and isolation.

When a symptom involves the head, it is important to see what part of the head is involved. Is it the male side or the female side? This will indicate a sense of separation from either a male or a female. If the brain is affected, it is clearly crown chakra tension, though it is important to consider also which part of the body or function is affected, and to describe it from the point of view that the person created it. If it is the forehead, it is more about the brow chakra and the person's thoughts and feelings about spirituality or religion.

Headache

A headache generally points to tensions in the crown chakra, and therefore with father and/or authority, or a sense of separation from someone. A headache at the level of the forehead, however, points more to brow chakra tensions and something happening in the person's thoughts and feelings about spirituality or religion, or not feeling seen as the person inside the body.

Hearing – See Deafness

Heart

Any symptom affecting the heart indicates tension in the heart chakra, and therefore in the parts of the person's consciousness concerning relationships and people close to their heart – partner, parent, brother or sister, son or daughter.

Heart Attack (Myocardial Infarction)

Myocardial infarction (MI) or acute myocardial infarction (AMI), commonly known as a heart attack, results from the interruption of blood supply to a part of the heart, causing heart cells to die. It is related to the heart chakra, and therefore the area of relationships, reflecting tensions or a shock concerning someone close to the person's heart (a partner, parent, sibling or child) with a decision that the resulting tension is unacceptable and that the person doesn't want to face life with that situation as it is.

Heartburn

Heartburn is a painful burning feeling in the chest or throat. It happens when stomach acid backs up into the oesophagus, the tube that carries food from the mouth to the stomach. It points to solar plexus tensions affecting the heart chakra – control issues or anger in the area of relationships. Sensations in the throat point to unexpressed anger.

Heart Chakra Tensions

The heart chakra is associated with the perceptions of love with people close to the person's heart – a partner, parent, sibling or child. Heart chakra tensions that can result in physical symptoms involving the heart or blood circulatory system, or the lungs, reflect tensions with someone close to the person at the time the symptom began.

Heart Valve Prolapse – See Barlow's Syndrome

Heaves

Heaves generally refers to vomiting or retching. Dry heaves is repetitive involuntary throwing up that is not accompanied by vomit. It reduces pulmonary function. Clinical signs may include coughing and bronchitis. The symptoms reflect tensions in the solar plexus chakra and a sense of something out of control, affecting the heart chakra and the perceptions of love with someone close.

Hemiplegia

Hemiplegia is a paralysis of one side of the body usually resulting from disease or injury to the motor centres of the brain or the nervous system. If it is the will side (right side in right-handed persons) the person has paralyzed their will in response to events in their life at the time the symptom began. If it was the emotional side, the person paralyzed their emotions, finding it difficult to deal with the emotions of what happened at that time. Because the nervous system is involved, and therefore the crown chakra, it may reflect tensions with father/authority, or a sense of separation from someone close.

Hepatitis

Hepatitis is swelling and inflammation of the liver, associated with the solar plexus chakra. It reflects strong anger about something happening in the person's life. Because it is considered highly contagious, it also points to crown chakra tensions, a sense of isolation, and separation from someone. The person feels alone and angry.

Hereditary Disorders – See Genetic Disorders

Hernia

A hernia is where an internal part of the body pushes through a weakness in the muscle or surrounding tissue wall. It points to pressure in one area coming out in another – anger suppressed about one thing that comes out or is expressed about something else that is not really the source of the anger.

Herniated Disc – See Disc Herniation

Herpes, Genital and otherwise

Herpes is an infection that is caused by the herpes simplex virus (HSV). Oral herpes causes cold sores around the mouth or face and reflects anger issues; the sores keep others from getting too close. Genital herpes affects the genitals, buttocks or anal area and thus is associated with anger about sexual issues or about root chakra issues (tensions at home, for example, or trust issues about sex). Other herpes infections can affect the eyes (anger about something the person sees), skin or other parts of the body.

Herpes Zoster – See Shingles

HHT (Hereditary Haemorrhagic Telangiectasia)

Osler–Weber–Rendu syndrome (OWR) is also known as hereditary haemorrhagic telangiectasia (HHT). The distinguishing feature of OWR is the occurrence of arteriovenous malformations (AVM). These are abnormal blood vessels in which blood flows directly from an artery into a vein without going through the capillaries. When large AVMs occur in critical organs like the brain, lung, liver or gastrointestinal tract, haemorrhage in these areas can become life threatening. Most HHT patients with gastrointestinal bleeding (GI) don't have symptoms but are anaemic or iron deficient. Anaemia can cause fatigue, shortness of breath, chest pain or light-headedness. Brain AVMs are present in approximately 10% of people with HHT and can cause haemorrhage leading to stroke and/or death, or to seizures.

As a disorder of the blood circulatory system, it is related to the heart chakra and thus perceptions of love, and the parts of the body affected reflect tensions in the chakras associated with those parts. In general, the person does not feel nourished by the love around them and feels isolated and insecure.

Hiatal (Hiatus) Hernia

Hiatal hernia is a condition in which part of the stomach sticks upward into the chest, through an opening in the diaphragm. It reflects solar plexus tensions affecting the heart chakra. It points to strong anger affecting the love in the area of relationships.

Hiccups, Hiccough

A hiccup is a sudden, involuntary contraction (spasm) of the diaphragm muscle. This spasm causes an intake of breath that is suddenly stopped by the closure of the vocal cords (glottis). This closure causes the characteristic 'hiccup' sound. As a muscle spasm, it reflects solar plexus tension affecting the intake of air, which reflects heart chakra tension with someone close – wanting to take in the air (love) but stopping it, through not communicating, due to the throat chakra tension.

High Blood Pressure – See Hypertension

Hips

The hip's primary function is to support the weight of the body in both standing and walking or running postures. The hip joints play the most important role in maintaining balance, and are related to the root chakra, and the parts of the person's consciousness related to security – money, home, job, mother and feeling supported. If there is tension on just one side, it can relate to trust in a male or in a female (depending on whether it is the male side – right side in right-handed people – or the female side), in terms of what was happening in the person's life when the symptom began.

Hirsutism

Hirsutism is a condition in which women develop male-pattern hair (such as facial hair). An excess of testosterone due to a medical condition is usually responsible. The person affected might feel that there is some advantage in being male, or a disadvantage in being female. Because it is also considered unattractive, it can be seen as discouraging sexual contact or relationships and thus it can reflect tensions in the sacral chakra related to sex, the heart chakra related to perceptions of love and/or the crown chakra, reflecting tensions with father/authority and/or a sense of separation or isolation at the time the symptom began.

Histiocytosis

Langerhans cell histiocytosis (also called histiocytosis X) primarily affects children. It is considered an autoimmune phenomenon and causes immune cells to overproduce and attack the body instead of fighting infection. The person's sense of protecting themselves from hurt in the area of relationships at the time the symptoms began is preventing them from letting in the love and feeling loved. It reflects heart chakra tensions at home.

HIV

HIV stands for human immunodeficiency virus. The virus attacks the immune system, and weakens the ability to fight infections and disease. AIDS is the final stage of HIV infection, when the body can no longer fight life-threatening infections. It is related to tensions in the heart chakra, and the person's perceptions of love. The person feels that their lifestyle separates them from someone they love, either because of their sexual preference or the use of socially unacceptable drugs, or the type of society in which they live. It is easier to find and practise love and acceptance in some societies than in others, where unfortunately conflict and control are more prevalent.

Hives

Hives (medically known as urticaria) are red, itchy, raised areas of skin that appear in varying shapes and sizes. They reflect issues of anger, and the part of the body affected reflects what the anger is about.

Hoarseness

Hoarseness refers to a difficulty making sounds when trying to speak. Vocal sounds may be weak, breathy, scratchy or husky. It reflects the person keeping him or herself from communicating or expressing something about which they do not feel good.

Hodgkin's Lymphoma

Hodgkin's lymphoma, also known as Hodgkin lymphoma and previously known as Hodgkin's disease, is a type of lymphoma, which is a cancer originating from white blood cells called lymphocytes. It typically affects the lymph system, related to the root chakra, though the fact that it originates from the white blood cells points to tensions in the area of relationships at home, and the person's defences going out of control – protecting themselves from those tensions with someone close. The fact that the spleen and/or liver are often affected points to unexpressed anger in the person with the symptom.

Hollow Back – See Lordosis

Hot Flushes

Characteristically, a hot flush is a sudden feeling of warmth and often a breakout of sweating usually confined to the upper half of the body (chest and up), neck, face and head. Because the element associated with the solar plexus chakra is fire, and sweating is related to the elimination system and therefore the root chakra, the experience can be seen as solar plexus energy emerging, and thus as being related to a change or reaffirmation of one's sense of identity, as when it is associated with menopause, and a sense of emerging confidence in the new sense of identity.

Human Papillomavirus (HPV)

Certain types of HPV can cause genital warts in both males and females. These types can also cause warts in the throat, a condition called recurrent respiratory papillomatosis or RRP. Other HPV types can cause normal cells in the body to turn abnormal, and might over time lead to cancer. These HPV types can cause cervical cancer and other, less common cancers, including cancers of the vulva, vagina, penis, anus and back of the throat (including the base of the tongue and tonsils).

Because HPV affects the sexual organs or other parts that can reflect other kinds of sexual activity, it can be related to ambivalent feelings in the area of sexuality (sacral chakra) as well as root chakra tensions – insecurity, possibly about sexuality. When the throat chakra is affected, resulting in difficulty breathing, it reflects tensions in the throat and heart chakras, and difficulty accepting love, possibly because of the tensions involving sex.

Hunchback – See Kyphosis

Huntington's Disease

Huntington's disease (HD) is a brain disorder that affects a person's ability to think, talk and move. The involuntary movements associated with the condition can look like jerky dancing. As a brain disorder, it is associated with crown chakra tensions with father/authority, or a sense of isolation or separation from someone close at the time the symptoms begin. The involuntary movements also imply a conflict between the solar plexus chakra, which is associated with the muscular system and ease of being, and the crown chakra, associated with the nervous system – and therefore a possible perceived conflict between what the person wants to do and how they think authority might feel about their way of being – or insecurity about doing 'the right thing' as an adult.

Symptoms involving the feet and legs point to root chakra tensions and insecurity as a perceptual filter, and the later symptoms affecting the heart and lungs point to heart chakra tensions, feeling unloved or perhaps undeserving of love, and possible anger at someone close to their heart.

If the eventual conclusion of the symptom is helplessness, the person has been making him or herself helpless in their consciousness, and thus soliciting being taken care of as a form of having love expressed to them, and in that way returning to an earlier period of their life in which they did not have to be responsible. The person may have also felt inadequate to the responsibilities of adulthood.

Hydrocele

A hydrocele is a pathological or abnormal accumulation of fluid in a body cavity. When there is an unusual emphasis of a body part, it is considered as an emphasis on that part in the person's consciousness. For example, a hydrocele testis is an accumulation of clear fluid in the scrotum, and would raise questions about what was happening in the person's consciousness in relation to sexuality or having children at that time.

Hydrocephalus

Hydrocephalus is a build-up of fluid inside the skull that leads to brain swelling. It reflects tension in the crown chakra and therefore in the person's relationship with their father or authority at that time. Symptoms can point to specific tensions in relation to authority/father. For example, loss of bladder control would point to fear or insecurity and root chakra tensions, vomiting would indicate control issues, muscle spasms would point to solar plexus chakra tensions about the person's sense of personal power.

Hyperactivity (ADHD)

Hyperactivity means too much muscle activity. This disorder makes it hard for a child to pay attention. Hyperactive behaviour usually refers to constant activity, being easily distracted, impulsiveness, inability to concentrate, aggressiveness and similar behaviours. The hyperactivity and aggression point to solar plexus tensions about power, control and/or freedom. The difficulty concentrating points to root chakra tensions, possible tensions at home, but can also be related to crown chakra tensions with father and authority, creating a sense of isolation and feeling separate from those around the person who is experiencing the symptom.

Hypercholesterolaemia

Hypercholesterolaemia is the presence of high levels of cholesterol in the blood. The eventual effects can be high blood pressure, heart symptoms or stroke, reflecting tensions in the heart chakra with someone close (partner, parent, sibling, child) and a sense of isolation or separation from someone close.

Hyperglycaemia

Hyperglycaemia is high blood sugar, and is generally associated with diabetes. The opposite condition, low blood sugar, is called hypoglycaemia. Diabetes is associated with the solar plexus chakra, and suppressed anger. The person is keeping sweetness from him/herself. When someone gets too close with sweetness, anger arises to keep the other person at a 'safe' distance. To carry glucose (blood sugar) into the cells as an energy supply, cells need help from insulin, a hormone made by the pancreas. Thus, when the pancreas does not handle the high blood sugar, the cells are not receiving the energy. This can relate to the person not allowing him/herself to be energized or nourished by the sweetness (the love) around them. See Diabetes.

Hypermetropia (Hyperopia) – See Far-sightedness

Hypersomnia

The word 'hypersomnia' means excessive sleep or sleepiness that interferes with everyday life. Hypersomnias are subdivided into primary, idiopathic hypersomnia (persistent sleepiness lasting more than three months without abnormal tendencies to enter REM sleep); and recurrent hypersomnia (recurrent episodes of completely reversible somnolence between two episodes). The sleepiness and lack of energy point to root chakra tensions about money, home and/or job. They also indicate a dissatisfaction in the person's life that they do not want to face. It is interesting then to ask what the person is 'tired of.'

Hypertension

Hypertension (HTN) or high blood pressure, sometimes called arterial hypertension, is a condition in which the blood pressure in the arteries is elevated. The blood circulatory system is associated with the heart chakra and the area of relationships in the person's life. The condition reflects tension or conflict with someone close to the person's heart – usually a partner, parent, sibling or child.

Hyperthyroidism

Hyperthyroidism is a condition in which the thyroid gland makes too much thyroid hormone. The condition is often referred to as an 'overactive thyroid.' The throat chakra is affected. The person is not expressing themselves naturally, but rather projecting an overactive persona to cover who they really are. Symptoms can include difficulty concentrating, fatigue and frequent bowel movements, and this points to tensions in the root chakra as well, not feeling safe to be who they really are.

See what was happening in this person's life when the symptom began, and what the conditions were that the person responded to by deciding that it was not okay to show themselves as they really are.

Hyperventilation

Hyperventilation can cause symptoms such as numbness or tingling in the hands, feet and lips, light-headedness, dizziness, headache, chest pain, slurred speech, nervous laughter and, sometimes, fainting. It can reflect tensions in the root chakra (insecurity or fear), crown chakra (sense of separation or isolation) and heart chakra (tensions with someone close).

Hypochondriasis

Hypochondria is a belief that physical symptoms are signs of a serious illness, even when there is no medical evidence to support the presence of an illness. People with hypochondria have an unrealistic fear of having a serious disease. There is tension in their root chakra, and they are experiencing fear as a perceptual filter. It is interesting to know when the symptom began, and relate it to tension in the root chakra parts of the person's life – money, home, job, mother.

The person seeks out reassurance from family, friends or healthcare providers on a regular basis. They feel better for a short time at most, and then begin to worry about the same symptoms, or about new symptoms; this can also be seen as a repetitive pattern designed to solicit love and attention from others, pointing to crown chakra tensions and feelings of being isolated.

Hypoglycaemia

Hypoglycaemia is a condition that occurs when blood sugar is too low. Symptoms may include double vision or blurry vision, fast or pounding heartbeat, feeling cranky or acting aggressive and headache. They point to tensions in the solar plexus chakra (anger) and crown chakra (feeling isolated). If blood sugar gets too low, the person may faint, have a seizure or go into a coma, reflecting tensions in the crown and root chakras, and feelings of isolation and insecurity, or a sense of separation from someone close at home. The person is soliciting love.

Hypogyneismus

Hypogyneismus or frigidity is the inability of a woman to obtain sexual satisfaction under otherwise appropriate circumstances. Either she has turned off her sacral chakra, which is related to sexuality, or she has tensions in her root chakra, governing security and trust. The gonads are controlled by the sacral chakra, and the openings to the body and thus the lips of the vagina are related to the root chakra, so if a woman is insecure, she might not function sexually; but it reflects more of a problem of insecurity or fear that when resolved can result in restored sexual function and an ability to experience orgasm.

Another consideration could be tensions in the heart chakra, related to the sense of touch and perceptions of love, and to the crown chakra, related to the connection with the father, and feelings of isolation and separation when it is closed. When the crown chakra is closed, the person may feel as though they are in a shell, not feeling contact with those around them. See also Frigidity.

Hypophyseal Adenoma – See Pituitary Cancer

Hypophyseal Nanism – See Dwarfism

Hypopituitarism

Hypopituitarism is a condition in which the pituitary gland does not produce normal amounts of some or all of its hormones. It is related to the brow chakra, the home of the spirit, the individualized consciousness in the physical body. Tensions in this area can point to the person not being happy about their gender, since one common symptom is decreased or absent sexual appetite. Headaches can point to crown chakra tensions with authority or a sense of separation and isolation, and fatigue can point to root chakra tensions and insecurity about money, home, job and mother.

Hypotension

Low blood pressure, or hypotension, occurs when blood pressure during and after each heartbeat is much lower than usual. This means the heart, brain and other parts of the body do not get enough blood. The blood circulatory system is associated with the heart chakra. Symptoms of hypotension may include confusion, dizziness, fainting, light-headedness, sleepiness and weakness and thus point to tensions in the root chakra. The combination points to heart chakra tensions with someone at home or lack of circulation of love at home.

Hypothyroidism

Hypothyroidism is a condition in which the thyroid gland does not make enough thyroid hormone. The thyroid gland is associated with the throat chakra and the person's ease of expression. They are not expressing themselves as they really are, not feeling safe to express their truth, holding themselves back from being who they really are. There may be tensions in the root chakra (security, home) resulting in related symptoms including insecurity, constipation, fatigue and joint pain.

Hysterectomy

A hysterectomy is an operation to remove a woman's uterus. Afterwards it is unlikely that the woman will have a child. From the point of view that we each create our reality, she is keeping herself from having a child – implying that she would like to have a child but has been giving herself reasons not to do so.

There is tension in her sacral chakra, and possibly her root chakra as well, reflecting tensions about money, home or job, or a sense of mistrust with a specific man or with men in general.

Ichthyosis Vulgaris – See Fishskin Disease

Icterus – See Jaundice

Ideopathic Hypersomnia – See Hypersomnia

Ileitis

Technically, ileitis is an inflammation of the ileum, the final portion of the small intestine, where it meets the colon or large intestine. A specific and more serious type of inflammation involving both the small and large intestines is known as regional ileitis, or Crohn's disease. A common symptom is pain in the lower right portion of the abdomen or around the navel. Other symptoms include loss of appetite, loss of weight, anaemia and diarrhoea, which may alternate with periods of constipation.

As an inflammation, the symptom reflects anger, and because it affects the elimination system, it points to tensions in the root chakra, concerned with security (money, home, job). Thus, it can point to anger about root chakra issues. The location of the pain also reflects tension on the will side of the sacral chakra, a conflict between the person's will and what their body is asking for, in terms of food and/or sex. See Crohn's Disease.

Ileocolitis – See Crohn's Disease

Immune System

The immune system is associated with the heart chakra and the thymus gland, and therefore with the person's perceptions of love. Symptoms directly affecting the immune system (HIV, AIDS) are associated with the perception that the person's lifestyle separates them from someone they love. Many other symptoms are also referred to as 'autoimmune', and thus can be said to relate ultimately to perceptions of love and feeling loved, though in those cases, see the part of the body affected in order to know the specific decisions the person made at the time the symptom began, and the specific tensions in their consciousness directly related to the symptom they experience.

Impetigo

Impetigo is considered a highly contagious bacterial infection of the surface layers of the skin, which causes sores and blisters, implying anger. The skin is associated with the solar plexus chakra, and therefore with issues of control and freedom, and what one shows the world (one's image), though when the skin is affected in a particular part of the body, see that part and the chakra associated with that part for more precision about the inner cause.

Because the symptom is considered so contagious, creating a sense of isolation, it points to crown chakra tensions with father or authority. Because it is most common in preschool and school-age children, see the relevance of the person's interaction with teachers and other children, or reasons for feeling very conspicuous.

Impotence

Erectile dysfunction, also known as impotence, is the inability to get and maintain an erection that is sufficient for satisfactory sexual intercourse. The person has turned off his sacral chakra, which is related to food and sex. Reasons for this might be found in other chakras, for example the root chakra if there is insecurity, solar plexus chakra if the person is holding anger or the heart chakra if there are tensions in the relationship.

Incontinence

Urinary incontinence is loss of bladder control, unintentional passing of urine. It points to weakness at the level of the root chakra, possibly tensions at home, and thus insecurity or fear as a perceptual filter.

Indigestion (Dyspepsia)

Indigestion (dyspepsia) is a vague feeling of discomfort in the upper belly or abdomen, sometimes in the chest, during or immediately after eating. This reflects tension in the solar plexus chakra (anger, or issues of control), or possibly tensions in the area of the heart chakra (relationships) if the discomfort is in the chest.

Infarction

Infarction is tissue death (necrosis) caused by a local lack of oxygen, due to an obstruction of the tissue's blood supply. See the part of the body affected for more details. For myocardial infarction (MI) or acute myocardial infarction (AMI), see Heart Attack.

Infection

Many human illnesses are caused by infection with either pathogenic (disease-causing) bacteria or viruses. Infection implies anger. For further details see the specific symptom, the function or part of the body affected and the chakra associated with that part or function.

Infectious Mononucleosis – See Mononucleosis

Infertility

Infertility is when a couple does not succeed in conceiving (getting pregnant) despite having regular unprotected sex. With the idea that everything begins in the consciousness, infertility begins with a decision not to have children. This can reflect an earlier decision not to be a parent, or it can be related to the conditions in the person's life at that time. The reason can be questions about the stability of the relationship, or questions of money or freedom, or how the life of the parent(s) might be affected by having a child.

Inflammation

Inflammation implies anger, and the part of the body affected reflects what the anger is about.

Inflammatory Bowel Disease (IBD)

Inflammatory bowel disease (IBD) is the name of a group of disorders in which the intestines (small and large intestines or bowels) become inflamed (red and swollen). This reflects anger about the root chakra parts of the person's life – money, home, job and/or the person's connection with their mother, depending on what was happening in the person's life when the symptom began.

Influenza

The symptoms of seasonal flu include fever, cough, headache, aching muscles and tiredness. Fever and cough reflect anger, headache reflects crown chakra tension (father/authority or a sense of isolation), aching muscles reflect solar plexus chakra tensions and the person immobilizing themselves with a perceived lack of power ('I can't...') and tiredness can reflect solar plexus tensions and root chakra tensions (tensions about money, home, job).

Ingrown Toenail

An ingrown toenail occurs when the edge of the nail grows down and into the skin of the toe. It reflects irritation, and the toe affected shows what the irritation is about. For details, see Toes.

Insect Bites

See the part of the body and/or the function affected as the result of the insect bites to understand the message of the symptom and why the person attracted the bites to that part of their body at that time in their life.

Insomnia

People who have insomnia have trouble falling asleep, staying asleep or both. As a result, they may get too little sleep or have poor-quality sleep. They may not feel refreshed when they wake up. Generally, people having difficulty sleeping either have a lot of excess energy, or are concerned about something happening in their life. Excess mental activity can be related to solar plexus tensions. For the other reasons, see what part of the person's life they have been concerned about in order to understand what needs to be resolved.

Intestinal Gas

Excessive intestinal gas reflects solar plexus activity and thus control or anger. The specific symptom of the intestinal gas reflects specific tensions. See Belching, Bloating, Flatulence.

Intestinal Parasites

Intestinal parasites are worms or protozoa, and represent something 'eating away' in the person's consciousness, bothering them about the root chakra parts of their life – money, home and job. Solar plexus symptoms of stomach pain, nausea or vomiting point to anger or a perceived lack of control over these parts of the person's life.

Intestines

In human anatomy, the intestine (or bowel) consists of two segments, the small intestine and the large intestine. Generally, the small intestine is related to the process of assimilation, and associated with the second (sacral) chakra, and the person's relationship with food and assimilating its nutrients, and the large intestine, the colon, is related more specifically to the root chakra and the process of elimination.

Part of the colon crosses the solar plexus chakra, and when this part, the transverse colon, is affected, it represents a combination of conditions involving the solar plexus chakra and the root chakra – thus, anger about root chakra issues (money, home and job). Since any part of this system relates to eventual elimination, any symptoms here reflect tension about root chakra issues in the person's life; though if there is physical discomfort, see which chakra is closest to the tension (if it is the second or third chakra) and consider tensions in that part of the person's consciousness in combination with or affecting the root chakra parts of the person's life.

Irritable Bowel Syndrome (IBS)

Irritable bowel syndrome (IBS) is a disorder that leads to abdominal pain and cramping, changes in bowel movements and other symptoms. IBS is not the same as inflammatory bowel disease (IBD), which includes Crohn's disease and ulcerative colitis. In IBS, the structure of the bowel is not abnormal. Symptomatically, though, the two conditions point to the same inner cause: anger (irritation) about the root chakra parts of the person's life – money, home, job and/or the person's connection with their mother, depending on what was happening in the person's life when the symptom began.

Irritation

Any irritation points to the person feeling irritated or angry about something, and the part of the body affected would point to what they feel irritated about, in terms of which chakra and function is affected, and what that indicates in terms of the part of the person's consciousness that has been holding tension.

Ischaemic Cardiomyopathy

Ischaemic cardiomyopathy is a term used to describe patients whose hearts can no longer pump enough blood to the rest of their bodies due to a narrowing of the small blood vessels that supply blood and oxygen to the heart. There are tensions in the person's heart chakra, and therefore in the area of relationships, tensions with someone close to the person's heart and the person not feeling the love from the other.

Itching

Itching can be related to irritation, and therefore to a sense of annoyance, with the part of the body affected showing what the annoyance is about, in terms of the chakra associated with that part of the body, and the function affected.

Jaundice

Jaundice, yellow skin, is often a sign of a problem with the liver, gallbladder or pancreas. These organs are associated with the solar plexus chakra and various ways of dealing with anger. The person is extremely angry about something happening in their life at the time the symptom began.

Jaw

Symptoms involving the jaw are associated with solar plexus chakra tension and anger, possibly about root chakra considerations (money, home, job) since the teeth and the gums are associated with the root chakra and can be affected by symptoms or tensions involving the jaw. Because jaw symptoms might also affect communication and thus the throat chakra, they can also represent anger that has been unexpressed.

Joints

In general, the joints are associated with the root chakra, when the symptom is systemic and affects much of the body. In that case symptoms relate to the root chakra parts of the person's life (money, home, job) and represent the person immobilizing him or herself through insecurity or fear. When the joints in a specific part of the body are affected, see the part of the body affected, and the possible effects of the symptom if allowed to proceed, for more precision about how the person has been immobilizing him or herself.

Kartegener's Syndrome

Kartegener's syndrome is a condition characterized by abnormalities in the protein structure of cilia, the tiny hair-like structures that are supposed to move mucus out of airways, and symptoms can include chronic bronchiectasis (a condition in which the lungs' airways are abnormally stretched and widened, caused by mucus blockage) and sinusitis, an inflammation of the air cavities within the passages of the nose, reflecting root chakra tensions about letting in the love, or difficulty letting in the love from the mother.

Keratitis

Keratitis is a condition where the cornea – the clear, round dome covering the eye's iris and pupil – becomes swollen or inflamed, making the eye red and painful and affecting vision. Keratitis is also known as corneal ulcer.

Irritation and inflammation imply anger. If it affects one eye, it reflects tension in the will or the emotions depending on whether it's the will eye (right eye in right-handed people) or the emotional eye. If it is the male eye it reflects anger toward a male; in the female eye it reflects tension with a female. When both eyes are affected, it creates a sense of isolation, pointing to crown chakra tensions with father/authority.

Keratoconus

Keratoconus is degeneration of the structure of the cornea. The cornea is the clear tissue covering the front of the eye. The shape of the cornea slowly changes from the normal round shape to a cone shape. There is tension in the solar plexus chakra, possibly in relation to father/authority (crown chakra issues).

Keratosis

Keratosis is a growth of keratin on the skin or on mucous membranes. A solar keratosis is the most common type, resulting from skin damaged by the sun over many years. It reflects crown chakra tension and a sense of isolation or sensitivity about how one appears to others, possibly within the context of conflict situations.

Kidney Abscess

A renal or kidney abscess is a pus-filled hole in a kidney that forms when the tissues of that kidney begin to break down due to a bacterial infection. It points to frustration about feeling helpless to do anything about a situation the person is not happy about, since the kidneys are located at the level of the solar plexus chakra but part of the elimination system associated with the root chakra – thus insecurity (root chakra) in the place of personal power (solar plexus chakra) – a perceived lack of personal power.

Kidney Disease – See Bright's Disease

Kidney Stones

Someone with kidney stones may experience back pains at the level of the kidneys, high blood pressure, vomiting and fever. The kidneys are located at the level of the solar plexus chakra but part of the elimination system associated with the root chakra – thus insecurity (root chakra) in the place of personal power (solar plexus chakra) – a perceived lack of personal power. The person feels helpless to change a situation in which they are unhappy. The high blood pressure would reflect tensions in the area of relationships, which could be the area the person is unhappy about, with a feeling of helplessness in the situation. Vomiting is seen as an issue of letting go of control. Fever represents anger.

Kidneys

The kidneys are located at the level of the solar plexus chakra but part of the elimination system associated with the root chakra – thus a symptom affecting the kidneys represents insecurity (root chakra) in the place of personal power (solar plexus chakra) – a perceived lack of personal power. It points to a sense of feeling helpless to do anything about a situation the person is not happy about. In children, the sense of helplessness can be their response to overprotective or overcontrolling parents, and not feeling they are capable of doing things for themselves.

Knees

The knees are related to the root chakra and thus to the parts of the person's life representing security – money, home and job. Tensions in the root chakra are experienced as insecurity or fear as a perceptual filter. In right-handed people the right knee is the male knee and can represent lack of trust in a male, or lack of trust in oneself as a male. Similarly, the female knee can represent trust in a female.

The polarity can also be described as the will knee and the emotional knee, with the will knee representing trust in one's will – having made a decision but not yet acting on it because of insecurity – and the emotional knee representing insecurity or mistrust in the foundations of one's emotions, likely due to emotional insecurity, emotional dependency or not standing on one's own two feet with regard to one's emotions. The person has also possibly been making decisions designed to hold on to someone rather than doing what is best for oneself.

In addition to the location of the symptom see the effect of the symptom, or what could be the effect of the symptom if it were allowed to get worse, and then describe it from the point of view that the person created it. If there is difficulty bending the knee, it can represent the person not wanting to bend their knee to someone – not wanting to feel subjugated or dominated – not putting their foot down about something – not insisting on doing something about a situation they have been unhappy about. If the effect of the symptom could be not to be able to walk, the person has been keeping him/herself from walking, giving themselves reasons to stay in an unhappy situation.

Kyphosis (Hunchback, Slouch, Scheuermann's Disease)

Kyphosis is a curving of the spine that causes a bowing or rounding of the back, which leads to a hunchback or slouching posture. The curvature is at the level of the thorax, and the shoulders rotate forward to 'protect' the area of the heart, pointing to sensitivities there, and the person not feeling loved.

Labyrinthitis

Labyrinthitis is an ear disorder that involves irritation and swelling (inflammation) of the inner ear. This interferes with one's ability to feel balanced and to hear. Vertigo reflects tension in the root chakra, and therefore in the parts of the person's life concerned with security – money, home, job. Difficulty hearing reflects tension in the throat chakra and indicates something the person does not want to hear, something the person has resistance to letting in. This symptom can thus reflect tensions at home, or insecurity as the person's response to something they have been hearing. There may also be nausea and vomiting, reflecting control issues, and ringing or other noises in the ears (tinnitus), reflecting tensions in the brow chakra and the person not listening to their inner voice and thus not living what is true for them.

Laryngitis

Laryngitis is swelling and irritation (inflammation) of the voice box (larynx) that is usually associated with hoarseness or loss of voice. The tension is in the throat chakra, and the person has been keeping him/herself from communicating or expressing something they are unhappy about. If there is difficulty breathing as well, this reflects tensions in the area of relationships and people close to the person's heart – usually a partner, parent, sibling or offspring.

Larynx

Any symptom affecting the larynx and thus the person's voice reflects difficulty in or resistance to communicating something the person was unhappy about at the time the symptom began.

Lazy Eye

A lazy eye is a childhood condition that occurs when the vision in one eye does not develop properly. If it is the male eye (right eye in right-handed people) it represents not seeing the male or tension with a male figure in the person's life. In children, the tension is likely to reflect tensions involving the person's father. If it is the female eye affected, it represents not seeing the female, or tensions with a woman or women in general in the person's life. The two eyes not working together points to a reaction to the male and the female not communicating, tensions between the parents.

Leber Atrophy or LHON

Leber hereditary optic neuropathy is considered an inherited form of vision loss. Although this condition usually begins in a person's teens or twenties, in rare cases it can appear in early childhood or later in adulthood. Men are thought to be affected much more often than women.

Although the condition is considered hereditary, it is important and relevant to see what was happening in the person's life at the time the symptom began, in terms of something the person was unhappy about and has had difficulty looking at or seeing. Because the vision loss results from the death of cells in the optic nerve that relays visual information from the eyes to the brain, it can reflect crown chakra tensions with father or authority, or a sense of separation from someone close.

With a variation known as LHON plus, there can be movement disorders, tremors and abnormalities of the electrical signals that control the heartbeat, again reflecting crown chakra tensions as well as heart chakra tensions with someone close. Additionally, some people with LHON develop features similar to multiple sclerosis, making themselves helpless before a strong authority.

Left Side of Body

In right-handed people, the left side of the body is the emotional side, or the female side, and this description is useful in understanding specific symptoms. Symptoms on the left side of the body therefore reflect emotional reactions to the situations in the person's life at the time the symptoms were discovered. When symptoms are generally more prevalent on the left side of the body, this can reflect the two sides of the brain not communicating, and thus a male and a female in the person's life not communicating. It commonly points to tensions between the person's mother and father, and the person's reaction to that situation. The left side of the body can then also point to tensions in the person's relationship with their mother.

Legs

The legs are related to the root chakra and thus the parts of the person's life representing security – money, home and job. Tensions in the root chakra are experienced as insecurity or fear as a perceptual filter. In right-handed people the right leg is the male leg and can represent something concerning trust in a male, or trust in oneself as a male. Similarly, the female leg can represent trust in a female. The polarity of right and left legs can also be described as the will leg and emotional leg, with the will leg representing trust in one's will – having made a decision but not yet acting on it because of insecurity – and the emotional leg, representing insecurity or mistrust in one's emotional being, likely due to emotional insecurity, emotional dependency, not standing on one's own two feet with regard to one's emotions and possibly making decisions designed to hold on to someone rather than doing what is best for oneself.

In addition to the location of the symptom, see the effect of the symptom, or what could be the effect of the symptom if it were allowed to get worse, and then describe it from the point of view that the person created it. If the effect of the symptom could be not to be able to walk, for example, it could be said that the person has been keeping him/herself from walking, giving him/herself reasons to stay in an unhappy situation.

Leprosy (Hansen's Disease)

Leprosy is a disease that damages the skin and nervous system, pointing to tensions in the solar plexus chakra and crown chakra related to these areas. Signs of leprosy are painless ulcers, skin lesions of flat, pale areas of skin and eye damage. Later, large ulcerations, loss of fingers, skin nodules and facial disfigurement may develop. Loss of pigment in the skin points to crown chakra tensions with father/authority, or a sense of separation and isolation. Loss of the fingers, related to the throat chakra, reflects the person giving themselves reasons not to let him/herself have the fulfilment of their goals, and the facial disfigurement reflects shame or guilt (the person hiding their face).

Leucopenia

A low white blood cell count, or leucopenia, is a decrease in disease-fighting cells (leucocytes) circulating in your blood. Because this is a basic function of the immune system, related to the thymus gland and the heart chakra, the symptom points to tensions in the area of relationships and the person not feeling loved, and vulnerable. This can also be the result of a closed crown chakra and a sense of separation from the person's father.

Leucorrhoea

Leucorrhoea is a vaginal discharge during pregnancy. It is thin, white, milky and mild-smelling and is considered normal, though it does tend to discourage sexual contact and certain sexual activities. For that reason, the person affected can examine their attitudes toward sex, particularly when pregnant, and resolve tensions there.

Leukaemia

Leukaemia is cancer of the white blood cells that normally help your body fight infection. The person's sensitivities and defences have gone out of control to the point where they have become life-threatening. Because it is a blood disorder, it points to the heart chakra and the person's perceptions of love. Protecting oneself from being hurt by those close to his or her heart has left the person feeling alone and isolated, and not wanting to face life with that condition. The person is not allowing him or herself to be nourished by the love around them. Because the blood cells form in the bone marrow, the symptom can also point to the root chakra, and therefore tensions with someone close at home.

Leukoderma

Leukoderma is a condition with localized loss of pigmentation of the skin. The pigment is associated with the crown chakra, and the symptom can result in a sense of conspicuous isolation, pointing to crown chakra tensions with father/authority.

Libido

Libido, or colloquially sex drive, is a person's overall sexual drive or desire for sexual activity, and is related to the sacral chakra. Symptoms affecting the libido are generally either addiction to sex or lack of interest in sex, depending on decisions made by the person involved. It is always a question of the individual state of balance for that person, and not determined by any external criteria.

Lichen Sclerosis

In women symptoms include white spots on the vulva and the skin shrinking and fusing, making sex uncomfortable. From the point of view that we each create our reality, it can be said that the person is keeping herself from having sex, giving herself reasons not to have sex. She may feel that she has not been seen for who she is, but rather as a sex object, and she may create the symptom in order to have others be obliged to relate to her in another way. There may be insecurity about her role as a woman and issues of trust with men, and because the location also points to the root chakra, she may also lack a sense of connection with her mother.

Men and boys can also be affected, with white spots on the foreskin; this can reflect tension in their relationship with their mother, insecurity about their role as a male in a male–female relationship and attitudes about functioning sexually as a man.

Ligaments

Ligaments are elastic bands of tissue that connect bones to each other and provide stability and strength for the joint. They are associated with the root chakra, though if the symptom involves a particular ligament or joint, see the part of the body affected, the chakra related to that part and the function affected. Thus, if a ligament in the knee is affected, see 'Knees' in this listing to understand the inner cause.

Limb Fractures

The skeleton and bones are associated with the root chakra, though if the symptom involves a particular bone or limb, see the part of the body affected, the chakra related to that part and the function affected, in order to understand the inner cause. Thus, for a broken arm, see 'Arms' in this listing, etc. Broken trust may be a consideration affecting that function.

Lipoma

A lipoma is a soft, fatty lump that grows under the skin. Although it is considered harmless, it represents something held in and not expressed, and the location of the lipoma and the chakra associated with that part reflects what it is that was not expressed.

Liposarcoma

Liposarcoma is a malignant tumour that arises in fat cells in deep soft tissue, such as that inside the thigh or in the retroperitoneum, the space between the peritoneum and the posterior (back) abdominal wall that contains especially the kidneys and associated structures, the pancreas and part of the aorta and inferior vena cava. Retroperitoneal tumours may present themselves with signs of weight loss, emaciation and abdominal pain. These tumours may also compress the kidney or ureter, leading to kidney failure.

Any malignancy is life-threatening, and therefore represents a reaction to a situation in the person's life that they found unacceptable at the time the symptom began or was discovered. Cancer represents something held in and not expressed, and the part of the body affected shows what was not being expressed. Thus, a liposarcoma in the thigh points to a root chakra shock – insecurity or fear with a male if on the right side in a right-handed person, or with a female if on the left side. In the retroperineum, it reflects tension in the chakra closest to the physical location of the symptom, on the will side (right side in a right-handed person) or an emotional shock if on the emotional side, with a sense of helplessness about resolving the situation, since possible effects might touch the kidneys.

Other symptoms can include fatigue (root chakra tensions about money, home and job), weight loss (sacral chakra tensions about food/sex, and the person not allowing themself to be nourished by the love around them), and nausea and vomiting (solar plexus tensions involving anger and control issues).

Lips

The inner cause of symptoms affecting the lips depends upon the function affected by the symptom.

For example, the lips are used for communication, and if this is the function affected, as with a swollen lip, it points to the person avoiding communication about something. An obvious and unattractive symptom (herpes, a cold sore) would discourage kissing and thus be designed to keep a prospective romantic or sexual partner at a distance.

Liver

The liver is associated with the solar plexus chakra, and is an organ said to store anger. Thus, when there is a symptom affecting the liver (cirrhosis or hepatitis, for example), the symptom reflects tension in the solar plexus chakra, and anger about something happening in the person's life at that time.

Liver Cirrhosis

Cirrhosis is scarring of the liver and poor liver function. The liver is associated with the solar plexus chakra, and therefore issues of power, control and freedom. Liver symptoms are associated with unreleased anger or frustration about an unhappy situation.

Lockjaw – See Tetanus

Long-sightedness – See Far-sightedness

Lordosis

Lordosis, also known as swayback or saddle back, is a condition in which the spine in the lower back has an excessive curvature. Lordosis can cause pain at the level of the root chakra or sacral chakra, reflecting tensions about security, or food and sex. If it affects the ability to move, the person has been immobilizing him or herself because of tensions in those areas.

Lou Gehrig's Disease – See Amyotrophic Lateral Sclerosis (ALS)

Low Blood Pressure – See Hypotension

Low Blood Sugar – See Hypoglycaemia

Low Energy

Low energy points to tensions in the root chakra parts of the person's life – money, home, job. What is the person 'tired of'?

Lumbago

Lumbago is a general term used to describe pain in the lumbar region, reflecting tension in the sacral chakra and therefore in the parts of the person's consciousness related to food and/or sex. There may sometimes be a tingling sensation or a feeling of numbness in the back, buttocks or down one or both legs, and this points to root chakra tensions, insecurities about the sacral chakra issues, or sacral chakra issues related to tensions in the person's home life.

Lung Cancer

The lungs are associated with the heart chakra and the area of relationships in the person's life. The element of air is also associated with the heart chakra, and a person's relationship with air reflects their relationship with love. One can then see the parallels with difficulty allowing it in, or difficulty expressing it.

Any form of cancer represents something held in and not expressed, and the part of the body affected shows what it is that is being held in and not expressed. With lung cancer and its association with the heart chakra, it represents difficult emotions held in and not expressed about something that happened in the person's life with someone close (partner, parent, sibling or child) at the time the symptom began or was discovered. Because the symptom can result in death, it shows that the person affected decided that the situation was unacceptable, and that he or she decided that they did not want to face life with that situation. They need to find a way of resolving that situation one way or another so that they have something to look forward to, something to live for.

Lungs

The lungs are associated with the heart chakra and the area of relationships in the person's life. Symptoms affecting the lungs affect the person's ability to breathe. The element of air is associated with the heart chakra, and a person's relationship with air reflects their relationship with love. One can then see the parallels with difficulty allowing it in, or difficulty expressing, in terms of what was happening in the person's life when the symptom began.

Lung Adenoma

Lung adenoma is a kind of lung cancer in which the cells might be considered benign, but because the symptom can eventually result in death, it can be considered malignant or life-threatening because of its location. See Lung Cancer, above.

Lupus Erythematosus

Systemic lupus erythematosus (SLE) is considered an autoimmune disorder that may affect the skin, joints, kidneys, brain and other organs. As an autoimmune disease, its original cause can be related to tension in the area of relationships, though considering the organ affected gives more details about the specific decisions made by the person at the time the symptom began. Difficulty with the joints, for example, points to root chakra tensions, possibly at home, and the person immobilizing him or herself because of insecurity.

A 'butterfly' rash over the cheeks and bridge of the nose affects about half of people with SLE, and this points to solar plexus tensions (anger) about root chakra tensions, possibly shame, or tensions at home. If the rash gets worse in sunlight, this reflects sensitivity to father or authority issues at home. The rash may also be widespread. See the organ or part of the body affected for further details.

Lyme Disease

Early symptoms of Lyme disease are similar to the flu and may include body-wide itching, reflecting irritation about something happening in the person's life; fever, indicating anger; headache, pointing to crown chakra tensions with father/authority or a sense of separation from someone close; light-headedness or fainting, reflecting root chakra tensions about money, home or job; muscle pain, pointing to a perceived lack of personal power, the person immobilizing themselves with 'I can't'; and stiff neck, reflecting the person not expressing or communicating. Loss of memory reflects root chakra tensions, anxiety, not feeling grounded and possible tensions at home. The heart can eventually be affected, and this would reflect tensions in the area of relationships.

Lymph System

The lymph system is considered part of the elimination system, and associated with the root chakra and therefore the parts of the person's life representing security – money, home, job, mother. If the lymph system is affected in a specific part of the body, it is considered as insecurity about the function represented by that part. Thus, the lymph system in the left underarm would represent insecurity about going for what would make the person happy in the area of relationships, since it would involve the throat and heart chakras, the closest ones to the symptom.

Lymphoedema

Lymphoedema is a condition in which the lymph system doesn't work well and there is water retention in the whole of the body or in particular parts. If the entire body is affected, it reflects tensions in the parts of the person's life related to the root chakra – money, home, job and/or mother. The elimination system, associated with the root chakra, is not functioning as it should. If the swelling affects specific parts, there is an emphasis on those parts, and it reflects insecurity about the functions associated with those parts. Thus, if it is the chest, associated with the heart chakra, the person might feel insecure in their relationships.

Lymphoma

Lymphoma is a type of cancer that begins in immune system cells called lymphocytes.

Abnormal lymphocytes collect in one or more lymph nodes or in lymph tissues such as the spleen or tonsils, and eventually they form a tumour. Because the lymph system is associated with the root chakra, symptoms in the lymph system can point to tensions at home, or insecurity about the function of the part affected. When the spleen or tonsils are affected, it represents unexpressed anger about a situation at home. See also Hodgkin's Lymphoma.

Macular Degeneration

Age-related macular degeneration (AMD) is a painless eye condition that leads to the gradual loss of central vision. The macula is a small area in the retina – the light-sensitive tissue lining the back of the eye. It is the part of the retina that is responsible for central vision, allowing one to see fine details clearly. When there is degeneration, central vision is affected.

In right-handed people, the right eye is considered the will eye, reflecting the person's willingness to see what they want, and the emotional eye is related to seeing what one feels. In our society, as one ages, they can have a tendency to consider themselves less important than others, and to focus less on what they want or feel. Vision is related to the solar plexus chakra, and ease of being.

If the macular degeneration begins in just one eye, it can represent a sense of separation from someone – a male if it is the right eye in right-handed people, a female if it is the other eye.

Malaria

Malaria is caused by a parasite that is passed from one human to another by the bite of infected mosquitoes. After infection, the parasites travel through the bloodstream to the liver, where they mature and release another form of parasite that then enters the bloodstream and infects red blood cells. The liver is associated with the solar plexus chakra, and anger.

The blood circulatory system is associated with the heart chakra, and when the red blood cells are affected, the person is not allowing him or herself to be nourished by the love around them.

Complications can include brain infection (crown chakra, sense of separation and isolation), kidney failure (root chakra tensions at the level of the solar plexus chakra, sense of helplessness about a situation the person is unhappy about), meningitis (crown chakra, possible tensions with authority), respiratory failure from fluid in the lungs (heart chakra and tensions with someone close) and rupture of the spleen leading to massive internal bleeding (solar plexus chakra and unexpressed anger)

Malignant Melanoma – See Melanoma

Manic-Depressive Disorder – See Bipolar Disorder

Marfan's Syndrome

Marfan's syndrome is a disorder of the connective tissue, the tissue that strengthens the body's structures. It affects the skeletal system, the cardiovascular system, eyes, and skin, reflecting tensions in the crown and root chakras, as well as the heart chakra. The person feels isolated, not feeling the love around them and feeling insecurity about that. It reflects tensions with the parents and reacting to not feeling their love.

Mastitis

Mastitis is a condition that causes a woman's breast tissue to become painful and inflamed. It usually occurs in women who are breastfeeding. Inflammation indicates anger and because the mother's ability to nurse may be affected, it may reflect her attitude toward breastfeeding or about facing the conditions of life with a new baby.

Mastoiditis

Mastoiditis is the result of an infection that extends to the air cells of the skull behind the ear. Symptoms can include fever (pointing to anger), headache (crown chakra, tension with father/authority, sense of isolation) and hearing loss (not wanting to hear something, anger about what one has been hearing).

Meares–Irlen Syndrome

Meares–Irlen syndrome (also known as scotopic sensitivity syndrome) is a form of visual stress that leads to difficulties with fine vision tasks such as reading. Attention and concentration difficulties indicate root chakra sensitivities (tensions at home or with mother), and headaches and sensitivities to light point to crown chakra tensions with father and authority. The possibility of epileptic seizures points to tensions between the root and crown chakras, or between the person's mother and father, as do the symptomatic similarities to dyslexia, where the two parts of the brain, the male and female parts, do not communicate. This is also reflected in difficulties with depth perception. All of this reflects the person's sensitivities to tensions or separation between their parents.

It is interesting that one proposed solution to the symptom is the use of green-tinted glasses. Green is the colour associated with the heart chakra and perceptions of love.

Measles

Measles is considered a highly contagious respiratory disease, though it is usually associated with the red-brown spotty rash that can affect the person. The respiratory system is associated with the heart chakra and perceptions of love, and the rash indicates anger. The symptom then, reflects anger with someone close to the person's heart. Not the same as German measles (rubella).

Melanoma

The vast majority of melanomas are from the skin but malignant melanomas have been described in nearly every organ of the body. Skin cancer represents sensitivities about one's appearance, how one feels about how they look to the world; and if other parts of the body are affected, see those parts to understand the inner cause. For example, if the nervous system is affected, that reflects crown chakra tensions, possibly concern about how one appears to authority or the father. Malignant melanomas, because they might be life-threatening, reflect tensions in a particular area with extreme sensitivity about how the situation might appear to others. See also Cancer.

Mellitus, Diabetes Mellitus – See Diabetes

Memory Loss – See Amnesia

Ménière's Disease

Ménière's disease affects the inner ear. It can cause vertigo, tinnitus, hearing loss and a feeling of pressure deep inside the ear. The vertigo reflects root chakra tensions, the hearing loss reflects resistance to hearing something and the tinnitus not listening to one's inner truth. The combination points to tensions at home at the time the symptom began.

Meningitis

Meningitis is a bacterial infection of the membranes covering the brain and spinal cord (meninges). Anything affecting the brain and/or nervous system reflects crown chakra tension in the relationship with father or authority. Headaches and sensitivity to light likewise reflect tension in the crown chakra. Other symptoms can include nausea and vomiting, reflecting anger and other solar plexus chakra tensions, as well as tension in the neck, reflecting throat chakra tension about something not expressed.

Meningoencephalitis

The layers of thin tissue that cover your brain are called meninges. An infection in these tissues is called meningitis. When your brain becomes inflamed or infected, the problem is called encephalitis. If both the meninges and the brain appear to be involved, the condition is called meningoencephalitis. Inflammation implies anger, and symptoms in the brain and nervous system are related to crown chakra tensions with father or authority. The symptom thus points to strong tensions with authority and anger about the situation, and a sense of isolation.

Menopausal Symptoms

If menopausal symptoms occur, they may include hot flushes, night sweats, pain during intercourse, increased anxiety or irritability and the need to urinate more often. These reflect tensions in the lower three chakras, and insecurity about sexuality and the person's shift in identity.

Menorrhagia

Menorrhagia is menstrual bleeding that lasts more than seven days, or is very heavy. It can interfere with sleep and daily activities. Blood loss from heavy periods can also lead to anaemia, causing symptoms such as fatigue and shortness of breath. Anaemia reflects the person not feeling nourished by the love around them. Fatigue points to root chakra tensions, and shortness of breath as well as blood loss reflects heart chakra tensions with someone close. The combination points to tensions with someone at home, and possible ambivalence about having a child.

Menstrual Problems

Menstruation problems may include amenorrhoea (absence of periods – not wanting to have a child at that time), dysmenorrhoea (painful periods – disappointment about not being pregnant, or feeling some disadvantage about being a woman) and menorrhagia (heavy periods – linked to ovarian cysts and/or uterine fibroids – reflecting ambivalence about having a child at that time.). Generally, mixed feelings about having children.

Mental Breakdown (Nervous Breakdown)

Mental breakdown (also known as a nervous breakdown) is a mental disorder that manifests mainly with features of depression or anxiety, reflecting tensions in the solar plexus chakra and root chakra. The person is depressed about something happening in their life, and because they feel they can do nothing about it. The anxiety reflects tension in the root chakra, and is therefore about money, home and/or work. Often this symptom is the effect of an unhappy love story that has gone out of control for the person affected. It can feel as though the world has come to an end, until the person succeeds in opening to acceptance of what is, thereby releasing the solar plexus tensions of control.

MERS Coronavirus

Middle East Respiratory Syndrome coronavirus (MERS) symptoms include renal (kidney) failure and severe acute pneumonia, fever, cough, expectoration and shortness of breath. It is often fatal. As a respiratory symptom, it reflects heart chakra tensions with someone close and difficulty letting in the love, and the fever and cough reflect anger. Renal failure reflects a sense of helplessness about the unhappy situation the person is in. As it affects only a certain region of the world, it raises questions about the conditions in the group consciousness that contributed to the situation, and the degree to which the individual accepted the beliefs and/or values that contributed to the symptom.

Mesothelioma

The tissue that lines your lungs, stomach, heart and other organs is called mesothelium. Mesothelioma is a tumour of that tissue. It usually starts in the lungs, but can also start in the abdomen or other organs. Since it most commonly affects the lungs, associated with the heart chakra, it represents tensions with someone close to the person's heart (partner, parent, sibling or child) at the time the symptom began. If other organs are affected, see those organs in this listing, and the chakra associated with those organs, for more precision about the inner cause.

Metrorrhagia

Bleeding more excessive than normal in menstruation or haemorrhage between two menstruations are symptoms of metrorrhagia. It reflects root chakra tensions (insecurity, fear) about pregnancy or about having a child.

Migraines

A migraine is a common type of headache that may occur along with symptoms such as nausea, vomiting or sensitivity to light, reflecting solar plexus chakra and crown chakra tensions with father/authority, and the person feeling out of control. In many people, a throbbing pain is felt on one side of the head only, and can reflect separation or isolation from a male or a female, depending on whether the pain is felt on the male (right) side or the female (left) side of the head.

Miscarriage

A miscarriage is the spontaneous loss of a foetus before the twentieth week of pregnancy. It may also be known as a 'spontaneous abortion'. It reflects ambivalence about having the child at that time. Consider the conditions in the person's life at that time, including questions about the stability of the couple.

Mitral Valve Prolapse – see Barlow's Syndrome

Mononucleosis (Glandular Fever)

Mononucleosis is a viral infection causing fever, sore throat and swollen lymph glands, especially in the neck. Known also as mono, it may begin slowly with fatigue, a general 'ill' feeling, headache and sore throat. This reflects tension in the root chakra (insecurity) and the throat chakra (unexpressed anger or frustration). A rash would be designed to keep others at a distance, and chest pain, shortness of breath or a cough can point to tensions in the heart chakra and therefore the area of relationships and the person not feeling loved. A headache and/or sensitivity to light reflects crown chakra tensions with father/authority and a sense of isolation. Because it most often occurs in adolescents, it can point to tensions in terms of discovering how to relate to members of the opposite sex.

Mood Swings

We use the term 'mood swings' to describe a reaction that isn't appropriate to the event that triggered it, and it can be one of the symptoms of menopause. See Menopausal Symptoms.

'Mood swing' can also be used to describe what happens with people described as 'manic depressive' or bipolar. See Bipolar Disorder.

Mosquito Bites – See Insect Bites

Motion Sickness

Motion sickness is a common problem in people travelling by car, train, plane and especially boat (seasickness). Motion sickness can start with a queasy feeling and cold sweats, leading to dizziness (root chakra tension – insecurity) and nausea and vomiting (solar plexus chakra tensions – letting go of control, feeling out of control).

Motor Neuron Disease – See Amyotrophic Lateral Sclerosis (ALS)

Mouth

The mouth has several functions, including eating, speaking and kissing, and the function affected would reflect the inner cause of the symptom. See the function affected, and then describe it from the point of view that the person created it, thus avoiding eating, avoiding expressing or communicating, avoiding kissing. Sores or irritation, such as herpes, reflect anger that has not been expressed, and also serve to keep others at a distance.

Mouth Ulcers – See Canker Sores

Mucoviscidosis – See Cystic Fibrosis

Mucus Colon (Mucous Colon)

Mucus in the stool is a common symptom of irritable bowel syndrome (IBS) and ulcerative colitis (a form of inflammatory bowel disease), and is seen to a lesser degree in Crohn's disease. All of these symptoms reflect tension or anger about the root chakra parts of the person's life – money, home and/or job.

Multiple Sclerosis

Affecting the nervous system as a whole, MS is linked to the crown chakra and the person's relationship with authority. By not standing up to authority the person is making him or herself helpless, talking to him or herself inside in a way that convinces them they cannot do what they want, cannot be who they really are, etc. The person is not standing on his or her own feet with regard to authority, and whoever is the authority for that person. Normally it is the father, but in some families, the mother is the father, i.e. she is the authority, the directing one. The 'authority' might also be a controlling partner. The person affected keeps him/herself from doing what they really want to do, in order to avoid a confrontation with authority. Sometimes this is done as an expression of love, sometimes as a fear of confrontation.

When the vision is affected, the person is keeping him or herself from seeing what they really want (right eye) and/or what they really feel (left eye), in order not to confront authority. It can also represent not seeing the male, tensions with men/a man (right eye) or not seeing the female, tensions with a woman or women in general (left eye); then it is interesting to see whether the 'authority' is a male or a female.

Mumps

Most commonly, mumps affects the throat, with swelling on one or both sides and pain, particularly when chewing. The throat chakra is therefore involved, pointing to something not expressed, usually anger, since the area is inflamed. It might be related to something that happened that is difficult for the person to swallow, in a metaphorical sense.

Since the person's ability to eat can be affected, as well as painful inflammation of the testicles in males, it can reflect tensions in the sacral chakra about food and/or sex or an emotional shock that the person reacted to by shutting down this chakra, not wanting to go into the emotion. The sacral chakra is associated with the emotional body, and the person's willingness to feel their emotions.

Fever is often present, which points to anger unexpressed, as do problems with the pancreas when that is an accompanying symptom.

Headaches, when present, point to crown chakra issues – either tensions with authority or a sense of separation from someone, feeling isolated.

Other symptoms of mumps can include dry mouth, sore face and/or ears and occasionally, in more serious cases, loss of voice, which again points to something not expressed or communicated.

Muscles, General

Muscles are associated with the solar plexus chakra, and with perceptions of power ('I can'). When the muscles are affected, there is a perceived lack of power ('I can't'). When the muscles in a specific part of the body are affected, this gives further details of the inner cause in terms of the chakra associated with that part of the body, and the function affected, described from the point of view that the person created it. Thus, muscles affected in the legs that could result in the person not being 'able' to walk would be described as the person keeping him or herself from walking.

Muscular Dystrophy

Muscular dystrophy (MD) is a disorder that weakens the muscles that help the body move. Because the effect is that the person becomes immobilized, it reflects the person immobilizing themselves in their inner dialogue, the way they have been talking to themselves with 'I can't'.
When it happens in children, it can point to possibly overprotective parents, and the child responding to these conditions by making him or herself dependent on being helped, in order to accept that expression of love.

Myalgic Encephalomyelitis (ME) – See Chronic Fatigue Syndrome (CFS)

Mycosis

A mycosis is a fungal infection. A fungus eats, so when there is a fungal infection, it can be seen as something 'eating away' at the person, bothering them in the background of their consciousness. The part of the body affected points to what it is. If it starts in the lungs, for example, it represents something eating away at the person, bothering them about someone close, preventing them from feeling the love with that person. See Fungus, Fungal Infections.

Mycosis Fungoides

Mycosis fungoides is a condition in which lymphocytes (a type of white blood cell) become malignant (cancerous) and affect the skin. As a blood disorder, it points to tensions in the heart chakra and the person's perceptions of love, and a situation in which the person's defences about being hurt in this area have become excessive. The fact that it affects the skin points to solar plexus chakra considerations in which the person may be concerned about how they appear to others, possibly within the context of the relationship.

Myelodysplastic Syndrome

Myelodysplastic syndrome (MDS) is a condition that affects the bone marrow and the blood cells it produces. Thus, it is a root chakra symptom (security, home) affecting a heart chakra function. It can turn into acute myeloid leukaemia, a type of cancer, so symptomatically it is seen as the person giving him/herself reasons not to allow themselves to be nourished by the love around them, and not feeling safe at home.

Myocardial Infarction

Myocardial infarction (MI) or acute myocardial infarction (AMI), commonly known as a heart attack, results from the interruption of blood supply to a part of the heart, causing heart cells to die. It is related to the heart chakra, and therefore the area of relationships, reflecting tensions or a shock concerning someone close to the person's heart (a partner, parent, sibling or child) with a decision that the resulting tension is unacceptable and that the person doesn't want to face life with that situation as it is.

Myopathy

Myopathy is a muscle disease with weakness occurring primarily in the muscles of the shoulders, upper arms, thighs and pelvis. The muscular system is associated with the solar plexus chakra, and thus issues of power. When the muscles are weak, the person does not own their power. Their thought processes tend more to 'I can't' rather than 'I can'. The person is making him/herself helpless and immobilized as the result of how they have been talking to themselves. When the legs are affected, there are root chakra tensions (insecurity) and the person is giving him/herself reasons to stay in an unhappy situation, possibly at home. The upper body weakness implies a resistance and a perceived insecurity about setting goals and seeing a positive future.

Myopia – See Near-sightedness

Myositis

Myositis means muscle inflammation, pointing to anger issues combined with a perceived lack of power and a sense of helplessness about the situation the person feels angry about. The muscles in general are associated with the solar plexus chakra. The part of the body affected (arms, chest, legs) can give further details.

Myositis Ossificans

Myositis ossificans is a bony growth or calcification that develops within a muscle following a contusion or strain. Bone is associated with the root chakra and issues of security. Muscles are associated with the solar plexus chakra and issues of power ('I can'). Thus, the symptom reflects insecurity affecting the person's sense of power. See the part of the body affected (arms, chest, legs) for further details.

Nail-Biting

Regular nail-biting that causes severe damage to the nail and surrounding skin can be considered a form of self-mutilation. Stress and boredom are the main reasons for nail-biting for most people. The habit is often a way to ease anxiety or to keep at least one part of the body occupied while the person feels bored, pointing to root chakra tensions, insecurity and not being present. The self-mutilation points to punishing oneself for reasons of shame or guilt, even though the shame or guilt may be without specific personal reason, but rather is because of closed crown chakra tensions, feeling isolated and thus not feeling the love around them, not feeling loved. When the nail-biting results in damage to the fingers, and the person has to hide their hands, that also points to shame or guilt and not feeling worthy of achieving their goals. If specific nails are involved, see 'Nails', below, for more precision.

Nails

The structure of the nails resembles nerve tissue, and if each finger were a person, the nail would represent the crown chakra. If a specific finger is involved, and the hands and arms are related to the throat chakra, the symptom is read from the level of the throat chakra. Thus, as described under 'Fingers', the nail on the index finger on the left or emotional hand would be read as having something to do with expressing (throat chakra) emotions (left side) about sacral chakra issues – food and/or sex (index finger) creating a sense of isolation (fingernail).

The toenails are read in a similar way. Thus, the nail on the big toe of the will foot (right foot for right-handed people) would be read as having something to do with insecurity (root chakra) about what the person wants (will side) concerning root chakra considerations – home (big toe) creating a sense of isolation (toenail).

Nanism – See Dwarfism

Narcolepsy

Narcolepsy is a neurological sleep disorder that causes excessive sleepiness and frequent daytime sleep attacks. As a neurological symptom it points to crown chakra tensions with father/authority or a sense of isolation. The periods of extreme drowsiness during the day and the person going out of his or her body points to root chakra tensions about money, home, job and/or the person not happy being where they are.

Nausea

Nausea is the feeling of having an urge to vomit. It represents tension in the solar plexus chakra, and can represent a feeling of things going out of control.

Near-sightedness

Near-sightedness is about seeing what is close better than seeing what is further away. The direction of attention is toward the inside, away from the outside, retreating inward away from a threatening world, contracting, a sense of hiding something inside, not wanting it to be visible. There is tension in the solar plexus chakra and also the root chakra, and the emotional perceptual filter is one of insecurity or fear.

Things must be held close to be seen clearly and comfortably. What the person wants or feels is experienced as more important to them than what others want or feel. An exceptional need for privacy may be experienced, a withdrawal from the world around them, a sense of being intimidated by their environment, a hiding inside.

The focus of thinking is forward, thinking of the future, of what might be, could be, etc., with fear or uncertainty as the emotional experience of that view. It is a preoccupation, keeping the individual from being totally present, in the here and now. The degree to which this is experienced is a matter of individual balance, and related to the degree of near-sightedness. Naturally, there may also be different compensations such as aggression to minimize the intimidation, or a forced extraversion to disguise the hiding within, but we are talking about the basis behind these outer actions.

What was happening in the person's life at the time the eyesight was affected gives a clue to why the person responded to the situation with insecurity and fear.

Neck

The neck in general is associated with the throat chakra, and therefore with expressing. The will side (right side in right-handed people) represents something about the person expressing what they want, and the emotional side represents expressing what they feel. It is interesting to hear how the person describes how they experience the symptom. 'Sore' or 'irritated' implies anger, 'pain in the neck' has another connotation about something or someone the person finds annoying. If the back of the neck is affected it might feel as though the person is carrying some burden, or some sense of responsibility for something. In any event, it is about something needing to be expressed.

Nephritis – See Bright's Disease

Nephrosis

Nephrosis is a degenerative disease, usually of a specific part of the kidney called the renal tubule. The kidneys are part of the elimination system and therefore related to the root chakra, but are located at the level of the solar plexus chakra. Symptoms affecting the kidneys reflect insecurity about power or a perceived lack of power. The person makes him/herself dependent, and feels helpless to do something about an unhappy situation.

Nerves

The nerves and the nervous system as a whole are related to the crown chakra, and therefore to the person's relationship with their biological father or authority, or a sense of separation from someone; isolation. If the nerves are affected in a particular part of the physical body, see what part of the body is affected, and which chakra and/or function is affected, and understand that in terms of what was happening in the person's life at the time the symptom began, there were crown chakra considerations that the person responded to in a stressed way that can be related to the symptom.

Nervous Breakdown – See Mental Breakdown

Nervous System

The nervous system as a whole is associated with the crown chakra, and therefore with the parts of the person's consciousness related to their experience with their biological father and/or authority, or a sense of separation from someone. Neurological disorders are therefore seen as the result of tensions with authority, and the effect of the symptom gives further details when described from the point of view that the person created them. Thus, multiple sclerosis, resulting in the person being 'unable' to stand, can be seen as the person not standing up to authority, making themselves helpless before authority. Disorders like Parkinson's disease that affect other systems, like the muscular system, can be seen as a conflict between the solar plexus chakra (muscles) and the crown chakra (nerves), implying that the person is ambivalent about owning their power before authority.

Nervous Tic – See Tics

Nervousness

Nervousness implies insecurity or fear, and is thus related to tensions in the root chakra, and in the parts of the person's life representing security – money, home, job, mother.

Nettle Rash – See Hives

Neuralgia

Neuralgia is a sharp, shocking pain that follows the path of a nerve and is due to irritation or damage to the nerve. Symptoms include increased sensitivity of the skin along the path of the damaged nerve, so that any touch or pressure is felt as pain, or numbness along the path of the nerve.

Symptoms involving the nervous system are associated with tensions in the crown chakra, and therefore with tensions with father/authority, or a sense of separation from someone. Because these symptoms involve sensitivity of the skin, they can also point to solar plexus chakra tensions involving issues of power, control or freedom. See the part of the body affected. When the trigeminal nerves in the face are affected, for example, creating facial pain, it can reflect that the person may have felt figuratively slapped in the face or deeply insulted at the time the symptom began.

Neuroblastoma

Neuroblastoma is a malignant (cancerous) tumour that develops from nerve tissue. It usually occurs in infants and children and can occur in many areas of the body. Because the nervous system is associated with the crown chakra, the symptom reflects tensions with the father or the authority figure at the time the symptom began. See the part of the body affected for further details of the specific tensions in the consciousness in response to the conditions at that time.

When the symptom begins before a child is born, it reflects the child's reaction to a sense of not feeling the contact with his/her father.

While cancer generally reflects a situation serious enough for the person to consider dying rather than continuing to live with the situation, neuroblastoma is one of the few human malignancies known to demonstrate spontaneous regression to a completely benign cellular appearance. Sometimes, in very young children, the cancer cells die without any cause and the tumour goes away on its own. In other cases, the cells sometimes mature on their own into normal ganglion cells and stop dividing. This reflects a resolution of the conditions the person reacted to when the symptom began.

Neuropathy

Neuropathy means nerve damage, pointing to crown chakra tensions with father and authority and/or a sense of isolation or separation from someone. Neuropathy is also the name given to a collection of disorders that occurs when nerves of the peripheral nervous system (the part of the nervous system outside of the brain and spinal cord) are damaged. The condition is generally referred to as peripheral neuropathy. Neuropathy usually causes pain and numbness in the hands and feet, reflecting root chakra tensions at home and insecurity about achieving one's goals.

Neuropathy can also occur with diabetes, pointing to anger with father/authority at the time the symptom began. See the part of the body and function affected for details of how the person reacted to the crown chakra tensions at the time the symptom began, and the decisions they made as a result.

Neurosis

A neurosis is an excessive and irrational anxiety or obsession. It reflects tension in the root chakra parts of the person's life – money, home, job, mother – and a fear response to the conditions in the person's life at the time the symptom began, with a possible generalization of the perceptual filter of fear to areas other than that which triggered the fear response.

Nodules

Nodules are growths that are considered generically like tumours, though they might be benign, and they therefore represent something held in and not expressed. The part of the body affected shows what it is that has been held in or not expressed. Thus, lung nodules would be associated with the heart chakra, and tensions with someone close in the area of relationships. Vocal cord nodules would be associated with the throat chakra, and something the person has kept him/herself from communicating or expressing. Consider the part of the body affected, the chakra associated with that part of the body and the function affected, in order to further understand the inner cause of the symptom, in terms of what was happening in the person's life at the time the symptom began.

Non-Hodgkin's Lymphoma

The non-Hodgkin's lymphomas are a group of blood cancers that include any kind of lymphoma except Hodgkin's lymphoma. Lymphomas are types of cancer derived from lymphocytes, a type of white blood cell. Because it affects the blood, the symptom points to tensions in the heart chakra and the area of relationships, and since the white blood cells are associated with the body's defences, the symptom reflects that the person's defences about being hurt in the area of relationships have become excessive to the point of being life-threatening. The fact that the cells are created in the bone marrow points to tensions in the root chakra, and therefore tensions with someone at home.

Normal Pressure Hydrocephalus

Normal Pressure Hydrocephalus (NPH) is a neurological condition, which normally occurs in adults aged fifty-five and older. As a neurological condition, it points to crown chakra tensions and a feeling of isolation. The feeling of feet glued to the floor, or difficulty walking, is the first symptom to appear in NPH, pointing to root chakra tensions at home. Later symptoms of memory loss and confusion also point to root chakra tensions about security, survival, trust and not feeling safe at home.

Nose

The nose and the sense of smell are related to the root chakra and therefore to the parts of the person's consciousness concerned with security, and that which represents security in the person's life – money, home, job, mother. Tensions in the root chakra are experienced as insecurity or fear. Cosmetic symptoms affecting the nose (blemishes, etc.) can point to a sense of shame or embarrassment (feeling like hiding one's face) or keeping others at a distance because of insecurity.

Nosebleed

Anything affecting the nose reflects root chakra tensions and a sense of insecurity or fear, and nosebleeds reflect not feeling safe, possibly not feeling safe at home.

Numbness

Described from the point of view that we each create our reality, numbness can represent the person keeping him/herself from feeling something, avoiding acknowledging an emotion about something; and the part of the body affected can point to further details in terms of decisions made in response to what was happening in the person's life at the time the symptom began.

Obesity

Because societal norms vary worldwide, obesity or being fat is not in itself considered a problem unless it is seen as 'excessive', unattractive or unhealthy. If it is considered unattractive, it reflects the person making him/herself unattractive; – and this points to sensitivities in the areas of relationships or sex, and thus not wanting to 'risk' being attractive because of the resulting unwelcome attention. That is why diets seldom work unless the individual resolves these sensitivities.

If there are perceived health risks, they point to specific inner causes. For example, heart difficulties indicate tensions in the area of relationships and the person's perceptions of love, while diabetes also indicates the individual holding others at a distance with anger, and thus also not feeling loved. Because the element associated with the heart chakra is air, and the person's relationship with air reflects their relationship with love, difficulty breathing points to difficulty letting in the love (not feeling loved) or difficulty expressing love. If someone's morbid obesity makes it difficult for him or her to move, the person has been immobilizing him/herself because of the sensitivities the symptom reflects.

Obsession

An obsession is a compulsive preoccupation with a fixed idea or an unwanted feeling or emotion, often accompanied by symptoms of anxiety. It reflects tension in the root chakra parts of the person's life (money, home, job) and can result in solar plexus tensions and therefore control issues involving the object of obsession.

Obsessive–Compulsive Disorder (OCD)

Obsessive–compulsive disorder is an anxiety disorder in which people have unwanted and repeated thoughts, feelings, ideas, sensations (obsessions) or behaviours that make them feel driven to do something (compulsions).

The anxiety points to root chakra tensions (insecurity in the area of money, home, job and tensions with mother), and the person's repetitive compulsive behaviour points to crown chakra tensions (father, authority and sense of isolation) in which they build their own reality in order to create more of a sense of security and feeling safe.

Oedema

Swelling caused by oedema commonly occurs in the hands, arms, ankles, legs and feet. It is usually linked to the venous or lymphatic systems, pointing to difficulties with the elimination system and therefore tensions in the root chakra parts of the person's life (money, home, job) and, if the arms and hands are affected, insecurity in the person's perceptions concerning setting goals.

Oesophageal Achalasia (Oesophageal Spasms)

Spasms of the oesophagus, which carries food from the mouth to the stomach, can be related to the person having difficulty 'swallowing' something, difficulty accepting some situation about which they have been unhappy. Achalasia is a problem with the nervous system in which the muscles of the oesophagus and the lower oesophageal sphincter (LES) don't work properly. The neurological association can point to crown chakra tensions with father/authority or a sense of separation from someone close.

Anxiety or panic attacks can also cause similar symptoms, and can be associated with root chakra tensions (about money, home and job). If there has been physical discomfort in the chest as the result of this symptom, it can also point to tensions in the area of relationships, tensions with someone close to the person's heart.

Oesophagitis

Oesophagitis is irritation or inflammation of the oesophagus, the tube that carries food from your throat to your stomach. Common symptoms include heartburn, pain when you swallow, chest pain (may be similar to the pain of a heart attack), a cough, nausea or vomiting and fever, all of which points to difficulty accepting a situation, likely about anger or solar plexus tensions with someone close.

Oesophagus

The oesophagus is the tube that carries food from your throat to your stomach. Symptoms affecting the oesophagus imply difficulty swallowing, difficulty accepting an unhappy situation. See Oesophagitis and Oesophageal Achalasia, above.

Oliguria

Oliguria is the low output of urine. It reflects root chakra tensions and insecurity in the areas of money, home and/or job.

Onyxis – See Ingrown Toenail

Orgasm, Lack of

A lack of orgasm reflects tension in the sacral chakra governing messages from the body to the person inside the body, and therefore the relationship with food and/or sex. A lack of orgasm can indicate the person's sexual activity not reflecting what their own body responds to, or the person not listening to his/her own sexual needs. It may also reflect tension in the root chakra, insecurity and the person not 'letting go' into the orgasm.

Osler's Disease (Osler–Weber–Rendu Syndrome) – See HHT

Osteoarthritis

Osteoarthritis (OA or degenerative arthritis) is a joint disease caused by cartilage loss in a joint. The main symptoms include pain and stiffness in the joints. The skeletal system and the joints in general are associated with the root chakra. The person has been immobilizing him/herself through insecurity or a lack of trust. See specific parts of the body affected for further details.

Osteomyelitis

Osteomyelitis is a bone infection, indicating root chakra tensions. See the specific part of the body affected for additional inner considerations. While the effects are often in the parts of the body associated with the root chakra (hips, legs, ankles, etc.), the arms can also be affected, pointing to throat chakra tensions and insecurity about the person going for their goals. Symptoms may include fever, reflecting anger about root chakra consider- ations (money, home, job, mother) at the time the symptom began.

Osteophytosis (Bone Spurs)

Osteophytosis is another name for bone spurs, outgrowths of bone tissue that form around damaged joints. The bones in general are associated with the root chakra, and therefore bone symptoms reflect insecurity. See the location of the symptom, then the symptom and the effect – calcification and immobilizing oneself through insecurity – in relation to the chakra closest to or related to the area affected. For example, lumbar (sacral chakra) osteophytosis would reflect the person immobilizing him/herself through insecurity in relation to food and/or sex. If it affects the neck, it reflects insecurity about expressing, and immobilizing oneself because of the insecurity about expressing.

Osteoporosis

Osteoporosis is a disease in which bones become fragile and more likely to fracture. The bone loses density, which measures the amount of calcium and minerals in the bone. The skeletal system is associated with the root chakra, and a sense of security. Therefore, the person affected is dealing with root chakra tensions, insecurity and increasing concern about root chakra considerations – money, home, job – and feeling more fragile, more vulnerable.

Osteosarcoma

Osteosarcoma is a malignant bone tumour that can develop in teenagers when the body is growing rapidly. It tends to occur in the bones of the shin (near the knee), thigh (near the knee) and upper arm (near the shoulder), though it can occur in any bone. The skeletal system is associated with the root chakra, and thus symptoms point to tensions at home or with the per- son's relationship with his/her mother, with insecurity or fear as a percep- tual filter. If one leg is affected, see if it is the male leg or the female leg, indicating issues of trust with a male or a female. Occurring in teenagers during periods of rapid growth, it points to insecurities about their future or about relating to members of the opposite sex, since those are significant factors in those stages. Cancer represents something held in or not expressed, and also indicates a significant shock in the person's life at the time the symptom began, pointing to a situation the person has not yet found a way to resolve. If the shoulder is affected, it points to ambivalence about going for a particular goal.

Otalgia (Earache)

Otalgia is ear pain. It hurts the person to hear something. On the will side (the right side in right-handed people) what they hear is contrary to what they want, and on the emotional side, it reflects an emotional reaction to what they are hearing, which is likely to be either conflict or something they might consider bad news.

Otitis

Otitis is a general term for inflammation or infection of the ear. It reflects anger (irritation, inflammation) about something the person has heard. On the will side (the right side in right-handed people) what they hear is contrary to what they want, and on the emotional side, it reflects an emotional reaction to what they are hearing, which can be either conflict or something they might consider bad news.

Ovarian Cyst, Cancer

An ovarian cyst is a fluid-filled sac that develops in an ovary. Both cysts and cancer represent something held in and not expressed, and when the ovaries are affected, it is in the area of sexuality or having children. In terms of the inner cause, the cancer represents more of a shock than with a cyst, with the person considering the problem so strong that they are not certain they want to face life with the situation as it is. If the cyst or cancer is on the will side (right side in right-handed people) there is conflict between what the body is asking for and the person's will, as if the body is saying, 'I want that' and the person's will is saying, 'I don't want you to want that.' If the conflict is on the emotional side, the person is dealing emotionally with what her body is asking for. See Ovaries, below.

Ovaries

Ovaries are associated with the sacral chakra, and with the person's sexuality or ability to have children, and therefore symptoms affecting the ovaries represent perceived conflicts in these areas. If the eventual possible effect of the symptom would be to have the ovary removed, and if it is described from the point of view that we each create our reality, it reflects the woman keeping herself from having children; although she may want to be a mother, she has been giving herself reasons not to do so at that time.

Overeating

Generally, overeating means eating more food than the body needs for energy or can comfortably eliminate. It represents a food addiction at the level of the sacral chakra, and while the person's relationship with food and sex (both associated with this chakra) generally parallel each other, if one is held back the other can escalate, and if the result is the person becoming obese, that can point to sensitivities in the area of sexuality or relationships. Thus, it is not about how much the person eats, but rather the possible effects of the overeating – making themselves unattractive.

Overweight

Obesity and being overweight are often considered synonymous, though obesity means having too much body fat, while being overweight means weighing too much. A person may be overweight from extra muscle, bone or water, as well as from having too much fat. Both terms mean that a person's weight is higher than what is thought to be healthy for his or her height. The specific health risk or perceived disadvantage points to the sensitivity in the person's consciousness. See Obesity.

Oxyuriasis – See Pinworms

Paget's Disease (Bone)

In people with Paget's disease, there is an abnormal breakdown of bone tissue, followed by abnormal bone formation. The new bone is bigger, but weaker and filled with new blood vessels. The disease may be in only one or two areas of the skeleton, or throughout the body. It often involves bones of the arms, collarbones, leg, pelvis, spine and skull. The skeletal system is associated with the root chakra, though here we must see the part of the body affected in order to understand the inner cause. If it affects the entire skeleton, or the legs or pelvis, it reflects tensions in the root chakra parts of the person's life – money, home, job, mother. If it affects the arms, or the collarbones, it is related to the throat chakra and the person's insecurity about going for their goals. If it affects the skull, it reflects tensions in the combination of root and crown chakras, either with the mother and father, or because of a sense of feeling isolated at home. If bone pain inhibits movement, the person has been immobilizing him/herself because of insecurity or fear.

Paget's Disease (Breast)

Paget's disease of the breast is a skin cancer that affects the nipple or surrounding aureole, and is almost always associated with an underlying malignancy, cancer of the breast; this points to tensions in the heart chakra and thus in the area of relationships. While the symptom is usually found in women beyond childbearing (and therefore nursing) age, the tensions may have something to do with tensions involving a son or daughter of the person affected.

Paget's Disease (Vulva, Penis, Scrotum)

Paget's disease of the vulva is a skin cancer that occurs predominantly in pre- or postmenopausal Caucasian women, and while it is located at the level of the root chakra, its presence can inhibit sexual activity, so it can represent insecurity about sexuality in relation to menopause. Often, women consider that menopause makes them less attractive to men, though men rarely consider that. When it affects the penis or scrotum in men, the inhibitory effect of the symptom may relate to insecurities involving sexuality or sexual activity.

Pain

Pain is a signal that something is wrong, and represents tension in the person's consciousness, with the part of the body affected pointing to further details about the reasons for the tension, considering the chakra associated with that part, and the function affected by the pain.

Painful Periods

Menstrual or period pain may be common but it is not normal, since it is not universal. It can point to disappointment at not being pregnant, or a perceived disadvantage to being a woman or functioning as an adult woman.

Palpitations

Palpitations are noticeable heartbeats that a person senses, usually because the beats are fast or irregular. Because they direct attention to the heart chakra, they can reflect tensions with someone close.

Palsy

Palsy is a medical term that refers to various types of paralysis, often accompanied by loss of feeling and uncontrolled body movements such as shaking. When the cause is neurological, it reflects crown chakra considerations or issues with authority, or a sense of separation from someone, and when the muscles are affected, it reflects solar plexus chakra considerations of power, control or freedom, perhaps the person feeling ambivalent about their actions because of possible conflict with authority. For the clearest understanding of the inner cause, see the part of the body affected, and the chakra and function associated with that part. Specific kinds of palsy have their own characteristics. See Bell's Palsy and Cerebral Palsy, for example.

Paludism – See Malaria

Pancarditis

Pancarditis is an inflammation of the entire heart: the pericardium, myocardium and endocardium. It reflects tension in the heart chakra and thus with someone close to the person's heart – a partner, parent, sibling or child.

Pancreas

The pancreas is a gland behind your stomach and in front of your spine. It produces juices that help break down food and hormones that help control blood sugar levels. It is associated with the solar plexus chakra and anger. When it is affected, the person is keeping sweetness from him/herself. When someone gets too close, offering sweetness, the person feels threatened in their power to be who they are and the anger then serves to keep others at a distance.

Pancreatitis

Pancreatitis is an inflammation of the pancreas, and represents extreme anger about something happening in the person's life at the time the symptom began, and reasons they have given themselves to keep others at a distance, possibly because of identifying with a role or their job rather than seeing themselves as the person in the role. See Pancreas.

Panic Attack

A panic attack, also called an anxiety attack, is a brief episode of intense anxiety that causes the physical sensations of fear. Symptoms and signs include a racing heartbeat, shaking, muscle tension, shortness of breath and chest pain. These point to tensions in the root chakra (money, home, job, mother), heart chakra (relationships) and solar plexus chakra (power, control, freedom), pointing to control issues or anger with someone close at home, creating fear about possible consequences.

Paraesthesia

Paraesthesia is an abnormal sensation of tingling, numbness or burning that is usually felt in the hands, feet, arms or legs, but can be felt anywhere. It can be caused by pressure on a nerve, pointing to possible crown chakra considerations (tensions with father, authority, sense of isolation), though it is important to see which part of the body is affected, and the chakra or function associated with that part of the body, and the effect of the symptom, for further details about the inner cause.

Paralysis

With paralysis, when described from the point of view that we each create our reality, the person has been paralyzing themselves, holding themselves back, immobilizing themselves, and the part of the body affected gives further detail in terms of the chakra associated with that part of the body, and the function affected.

Paranoia

Paranoia is about seeing patterns in seemingly unrelated events all coming together as an apparent conspiracy. It points to throat chakra perceptions of interacting with another level of consciousness, combined with root chakra tensions creating an emotional perceptual filter of insecurity or fear, resulting in a perception of a perceived conspiracy. An accompanying sense of isolation can also point to closed crown chakra tensions with father or authority, or a sense of separation from someone at the time the symptom began.

It should be mentioned that when the filter of fear is released, the same perception of patterns of seemingly unrelated events all coming together as an apparent conspiracy can have a positive aspect, where the universe is perceived as a benevolent entity working on the person's behalf, intent on their happiness: positive paranoia, also known as grace.

Parasites

Parasites are living things that use other living things – like your body – for food and a place to live. Parasitic diseases can cause mild discomfort or be deadly. Parasites represent something 'eating away' at the person in their consciousness, though to have a fuller understanding of the specific inner cause, it is important to see what part of the body or function in the body is affected, and the chakra associated with that part of the body.

Paresis

Paresis is a slight or partial paralysis. See the part of the body affected for details of how the person has been paralyzing him/herself, holding him/herself back from acting or doing something. When it is due to destruction of or damage to brain tissue, it reflects tension with father/authority.

Parinaud Oculoglandular Syndrome (POS)

Parinaud oculoglandular syndrome is an eye problem caused by an infection, and is similar to conjunctivitis (pink-eye). It usually affects only one eye and occurs with swollen lymph nodes and an illness with a fever, reflecting insecurity and anger with a male if the male eye is affected (right eye in right-handed people) or with a female if it is the female eye affected.

Parinaud's Syndrome

Parinaud's syndrome is an eye disorder in which the person is unable to look up. Because it is caused by a brain disorder it is related to crown chakra tensions with father/authority.

Parkinson's Disease

Parkinson's disease is a disorder of the brain that leads to shaking (tremors) and difficulty with muscles involved with walking, movement and coordination. There is a conflict between the crown chakra (nerves) and the solar plexus chakra (muscles), thus between authority and the person's sense of personal power. The person feels ambivalent about going for what they want, for concerns that it might not be okay with authority.

Parotiditis (Parotitis)

Parotitis is an inflammation of one or both parotid glands, the major salivary glands located on either side of the face. It reflects throat chakra tensions. The person has difficulty communicating about something they are not happy about in their life. On the will side (right side in right-handed people) it is difficulty expressing what they want. On the emotional side, it reflects difficulty expressing feelings. For infectious or epidemic parotitis see Mumps.

Pellagra

Pellagra results from a deficiency of niacin (vitamin B3). Symptoms include generalised weakness and diarrhoea, pointing to root chakra tensions, likely about survival and home tensions. Irritability, aggression and vomiting as well as skin sensitivity point to solar plexus chakra tensions and feeling out of control, while abdominal pain and loss of appetite reflect sacral chakra tensions, likely about food. Seizures and dementia that may present as depression, followed by memory deficits and hallucinations or psychosis, may occur, reflecting crown chakra tensions with authority. The person is shutting down in response to intense conditions in their life at the time the symptom began.

Pelvic Inflammatory Disease (PID)

Pelvic inflammatory disease is a bacterial infection of the female upper genital tract, including the womb, Fallopian tubes and ovaries. Symptoms include pain around the pelvis or lower abdomen, discomfort or pain during sex that is felt deep inside the pelvis, bleeding between periods and after sex, unusual vaginal discharge, especially if it is yellow or green, and fever and vomiting, all pointing to anger and tension about sex and having children at that time, possibly due to tensions with the person's partner.

Pelvis

Symptoms affecting the pelvis reflect root chakra tensions about home, and not feeling supported. If mobility is affected, the person is keeping him/herself from walking, or giving him/herself reasons to stay in an unhappy situation because of insecurity. If the will side is affected (right side in right-handed people) the person is ambivalent about or not insisting on doing what they want. If the emotional side is affected, it implies emotional dependency. If the right/left polarity is seen as male/female, it can reflect tensions or mistrust with a male or a female in the person's life at the time the symptom began.

Pemphigus Vulgaris

Pemphigus vulgaris is considered an autoimmune disorder that involves blistering and sores of the skin and mucous membranes. About 50% of people with this condition first develop painful blisters and sores in the mouth, followed by skin blisters that may be located in the mouth, on the scalp, trunk or other skin areas. Blisters imply anger, probably unexpressed, as they affect the mouth. On the scalp, they point to crown chakra tensions (anger at authority or about a sense of separation from someone). On the trunk, they point to tensions in the area of relationships, anger with people close to the person's heart. Described as an autoimmune disorder, the symptom in general points to the tensions and anger with someone close to the person affected.

Penis

Since the penis has a role in elimination as well as sexuality, symptoms that affect the penis reflect tensions in one or both of these areas involving the bottom two chakras. They reflect tensions in the root chakra parts of the person's life (money, home, job) and/or insecurities about functioning as a sexual male.

Peptic Ulcer

A peptic ulcer is a defect in the lining of the stomach or the first part of the small intestine, an area called the duodenum. A peptic ulcer in the stomach is called a gastric ulcer. An ulcer in the duodenum is called a duodenal ulcer. The stomach is associated with the solar plexus chakra, and issues of power, control and/or freedom. Ulcers imply anger. Therefore the symptom points to anger, possibly about control issues. Symptoms that include bloody stools or fatigue point to root chakra tensions at home or at work, and chest pains reflect tensions in the heart chakra, and thus with people close to the person's heart.

Pericarditis

Pericarditis is inflammation (swelling) of the pericardium, which is the fluid-filled sac that surrounds your heart. Inflammation implies anger, and any symptom affecting the heart reflects tensions with someone close to the person. Thus, this symptom reflects anger with someone close to the person's heart.

Periodontitis, Periodontal Disease

Periodontitis means inflammation around the tooth; it is a gum infection that damages the soft tissue and bone that supports the tooth. The teeth and gums are related to the root chakra. Inflammation implies anger; thus, this symptom represents anger or tensions in the root chakra parts of the person's life, and therefore to the parts of the person's consciousness dealing with security and those things that represent security – money, home, job. The possibility of tooth loss points to a weak root chakra; a deteriorated sense of security and lack of roots.

Peritonitis

Peritonitis is an inflammation of the peritoneum, the thin tissue that lines the inner wall of the abdomen and covers most of the abdominal organs. The first symptoms of peritonitis are poor appetite and nausea, and a dull abdominal ache that quickly turns into persistent, severe abdominal pain, which is worsened by any movement. Additional symptoms include vomiting, fever and difficulty passing urine. The combination reflects solar plexus and root chakra tensions, thus anger and insecurity about the root chakra parts of the person's life – money, home, job.

Peritonsillar Abscess (Quinsy)

A peritonsillar abscess is pus that has collected in the space between a tonsil and the wall of the mouth, creating a large abscess. The patient will be unable to open his/her mouth and will almost always have an altered 'hot potato' voice with a fever. The symptom points to unexpressed anger.

Perspiration, Excessive

Excessive perspiration reflects insecurity and root chakra tensions about money, home, job and/or mother, since perspiration is considered a function of the elimination system associated with the root chakra.

Pertussis – See Whooping Cough

Pes Valgus

Pes valgus is an outward-turning deformity of the foot. If it affects the male foot (right foot in right-handed people) it points to a lack of contact or a sense of separation from a male, and if the other foot, from a female. When it happens in children, it points to the child's sense of disconnection from his or her father or mother.

Petit Mal (Epilepsy)

A 'petit mal seizure' is the term commonly given to a staring spell, most commonly called an 'absence seizure', a letting go at the level of the root chakra and not being present as the result of activity in the crown chakra. It is a brief (usually less than fifteen seconds) disturbance of brain function due to abnormal electrical activity in the brain, which is associated with tensions in the crown chakra, and therefore tension in the person's relationship with father and/or authority. Not being present reflects tension in the root chakra, and therefore t tensions in the person's relationship with his/her mother, or not feeling safe. The combination raises questions about events or feelings to do with the father causing a sense of letting go with the mother, and therefore a possible reaction to the sense of separation between the person's parents. See Epilepsy.

Peyronie's Disease (Chronic Inflammation of the Tunica Albuginea/CITA)

Peyronie's disease is a connective tissue disorder involving the growth of fibrous plaques in the soft tissue of the penis. Specifically, scar tissue forms, causing pain, abnormal curvature, erectile dysfunction, indentation, loss of girth and shortening. Because the penis has functions related to the elimination system (root chakra) and sexuality (sacral chakra), it reflects insecurity affecting sexual function, or repeated tensions (scars) at home (root chakra) or with a female partner, affecting the person's inclination to have sex.

Pfeiffer's Disease – See Mononucleosis

Pharyngitis

Pharyngitis is a sore throat caused by inflammation of the back of the throat. This reflects tensions in the throat chakra, and unexpressed anger.

Phimosis

Phimosis is a constriction of the opening of the foreskin so that it cannot be drawn back over the tip of the penis. It can reflect root chakra tensions with home and/or mother, and since the retraction would be important for adult sexual functioning, possible ambivalence about functioning as an adult male – possibly reflecting a reaction to tensions between the person's parents.

Phlebitis

Phlebitis is an inflammation of a vein, usually in the legs, which are associated with the root chakra. The blood circulatory system is associated with the heart chakra. Thus, the symptom can reflect anger or tensions (inflammation) with the mother, affecting the circulation of love with the mother, or tensions affecting the circulation of love at home. If it affects the arms or neck, it affects throat chakra functions, and can reflect heart chakra tensions with someone close giving the person reasons not to go for their goals.

Phobia

A phobia is an irrational and excessive fear of an object or situation, thus reflecting root chakra tensions about something happening in the person's life when the symptom began, and that may have become more generalized as a filter of fear affecting other areas. If the phobia affects breathing it can reflect heart chakra functions as well, and may also be the result of a sense of isolation related to closing of the crown chakra and thus a sense of separation from someone or tensions with the person's father.

Piles – See Haemorrhoids

Pilonodial Cyst

A pilonodial cyst is a cyst or abscess at the end of the tailbone, at the level of the root chakra. A cyst represents something held in and not expressed, and an abscess points to anger about something. Thus, this symptom points to anger held in and not expressed about the root chakra parts of the person's life (money, home, job, mother) in terms of what was happening in the person's life at the time the symptom began.

Pimples

Pimples occur when the oil-producing glands at the base of the hair follicles become overactive. The most vulnerable parts of the body are the face, back, chest and shoulders. They can reflect anger or solar plexus energy (considerations of power, control or freedom), and the location indicates further precision about the inner cause. On the face, the pimples tend to keep away possible partners for sex or relationships, and therefore reflect a sensitivity about not wanting to lose oneself in these areas. On the shoulders they represent unexpressed anger and/or solar plexus considerations (possibly about freedom) affecting the person going for their goals. On the chest and back they represent anger and solar plexus energy in the area of relationships.

Pineal Gland

The pineal gland is a pinecone-shaped gland of the endocrine system that produces several important hormones including melatonin, a hormone that regulates sleep cycles in response to light. Symptoms affecting the pineal gland or its functions reflect crown chakra tensions with the person's father or authority, or a sense of separation from someone.

Pinguecula

A pinguecula is a non-cancerous growth of the clear, thin tissue (conjunctiva) that lies over the white part of the eye and the condition is thought to be caused by ultraviolet light. Often, sensitivity to light reflects crown chakra tensions with father/authority. Because one possible effect can be dry eyes, the person has been keeping him/herself from crying, having difficulty acknowledging being unhappy about something happening in their life, possibly in relation to the person's father or authority. If only one eye is affected it can represent tension with a male (right eye in right-handed people) or a female.

Pink-eye

Conjunctivitis (also called pink-eye or Madras eye) is inflammation of the conjunctiva (the outermost layer of the eye and the inner surface of the eyelids). The person feels irritated or angry about something, and would like to avoid looking at that situation. If it is the will eye (right eye in right-handed people), it can involve something contrary to what the person wants, or tension with a male, and if it is the other eye, the emotional eye, it would be more of an emotional reaction or tension with a female.

Viral conjunctivitis is often associated with an infection of the upper respiratory tract, a common cold and/or a sore throat, and this points to tensions in the area of the heart chakra (relationships, perceptions of love) and the throat chakra (unexpressed anger).

Pinworms

Oxyuriasis (enterobiasis) is an infestation with pinworms, white parasitic worms about the length of a staple that can live in the large intestine and/or the rectum of humans. They reflect something 'eating away' at the person's sense of security, a background tension in the root chakra parts of the person's life – money, home and/or job. Thus, they reflect insecurity about something or possible tensions at home. See Intestinal Parasites.

Pituitary Cancer

The hypophysis, or pituitary gland, secretes hormones and is associated with the brow chakra. Tumours of this organ (called adenomas) are usually benign and half of them produce excess levels of hormones. Pituitary cancer or hypophyseal adenomas cause symptoms such as headaches, hydrocephalus, restricted field of vision, weakened vision and even blindness, reflecting crown chakra tensions and a sense of isolation, possibly due to ambivalence about the sexual role. Disturbance of the normal physiological function of the hypophysis can result in hormonal disorders, again reflecting ambivalence about the person's gender, and excess hormone production. See Acromegaly, Cushing's Disease and Prolactinoma.

Pituitary Gland

The pituitary gland is considered the master controller of the endocrine system, and is associated with the brow chakra and the level of consciousness known as the spirit, or in the Western traditions, the unconscious or subconscious. It controls growth, and since it is at this level that one is either a male or female individualized consciousness, disorders of the pituitary gland can point to tensions in the consciousness about one's assigned sexual role, or deep tensions in the consciousness about the events in the person's life at the time the symptom began.

Plantar Warts

Plantar warts are non-cancerous skin growths on the sole of the foot. Because they can affect walking if allowed to grow, they can reflect an unpleasant situation the person may have been keeping him/herself from walking away from. The symptom may also represent questions of trust in a male or in a female, depending on whether the male foot (right foot in right-handed people) or the female foot is affected, in terms of what was happening in the person's life when the symptom began.

Platelets

Platelets are cells that circulate in the blood and clot to keep us from bleeding. Symptoms that affect these cells thus result in excessive bleeding, reflecting excessive sensitivity in the area affected. See Haemorrhage.

Plates Sclerosis – See End Plate Sclerosis

Pleurisy (Pleuritis)

Pleurisy (also known as pleuritis) is an inflammation of the pleura, the lining surrounding the lungs. Symptoms include chest pain and difficulty breathing, and thus point to heart chakra tensions and anger with someone close.

PMS (Premenstrual Syndrome)

Premenstrual syndrome (PMS) is a collection of emotional symptoms, with or without physical symptoms, related to a woman's menstrual cycle. They reflect tensions in her consciousness about functioning as a woman, or about menstruating – having periods.

Physical symptoms may include pain and discomfort at the level of the sacral chakra, thus tensions about sex or not being pregnant; headaches, pointing to crown chakra tensions and a sense of separation or isolation, perhaps feeling judged for having the period; muscle and joint pain, pointing to root chakra tensions, feeling insecure and immobilized; breast tenderness, with possible sensitivity about not being pregnant; dizziness or tiredness, pointing to root chakra tensions and insecurity; and nausea, pointing to feeling a loss of control.

Psychological symptoms may include feeling irritable or angry, or depressed, both reflecting solar plexus tensions; or anxiety, confusion and forgetfulness, or difficulty concentrating, reflecting root chakra tensions. Loss of libido or loss of appetite would reflect shutting down the sacral chakra, possibly because of sensitivity about sex or the menstrual cycle.

The sacral chakra is associated with the menstrual cycle, and also with the emotional body and the person's willingness to feel their emotions. Increased sensitivity during the menstrual cycle allows emotional tensions to come to the surface that may have been held back in the person's everyday life.

Pneumonia

Pneumonia is a lung infection that may result in a cough, a fever and difficulty breathing. The lungs are associated with the heart chakra and the area of relationships, as well as the element of air, and a person's relationship with air reflects their relationship with love. Thus, the symptom reflects tension in the area of the heart chakra and anger with someone close to the person's heart.

Poison Ivy, Oak, Sumac Rash

Poison ivy, oak, and sumac are plants that commonly cause an allergic skin reaction to the oils they produce. The result is typically an itching, red rash with bumps or blisters. The irritation implies anger, and the part of the body affected can provide further details of the inner cause. For example, on the hands it could represent the person not allowing him/herself to have the fulfilment of their goals, and blisters there can point to anger blocking that process. If the blisters are on the legs or feet, the symptom represents anger about root chakra considerations – money, home, job.

Polio/Poliomyelitis

Polio is a viral disease that may affect the spinal cord, causing muscle weakness and paralysis, most commonly of the legs. Paralysis of the muscles of breathing and swallowing can be fatal. The nervous system and spinal cord are associated with the crown chakra, and the person's sense of connection with father and authority. Symptoms affecting the legs are associated with the root chakra and insecurity. Thus, the symptom reflects the person not standing up to authority – being insecure in the face of authority/father, possibly not feeling safe at home because of those tensions. Difficulty breathing reflects difficulty letting in the love (heart chakra) – not feeling loved. Difficulty swallowing reflects something difficult for the person to 'swallow,' metaphorically – difficult for them to accept.

Polycystic Ovary Syndrome (PCOS)

Polycystic ovary syndrome is a problem in which there are tiny cysts on the ovaries, and hormones out of balance. It can cause problems with getting pregnant. Cysts represent something held in and not expressed, and the part of the body reflects what it is. In this case, it is about sex or having children, since those are the functions of the ovaries. The woman would like to have children, but is giving herself reasons not to do so at that time. If it is not treated, over time it can lead to or be followed by diabetes and heart disease, reflecting solar plexus tensions of anger and heart chakra tensions with someone close.

Other common symptoms such as acne and weight gain reflect keeping a partner at a distance and discouraging physical and sexual contact.

Polymyalgia Rheumatica (PMR)

Polymyalgia rheumatica (PMR) is a condition that causes pain, stiffness and inflammation in the muscles around the shoulders, neck and hips. This reflects tensions in the throat and root chakras, or unexpressed anger about root chakra security considerations (money, home and job) and possible insecurity about expressing anger.

Polyneuropathy

Neuropathy means a disease of, or damage to, nerves. When it occurs outside of the brain or spinal cord, it is called a peripheral neuropathy. Mononeuropathy means one nerve is involved. Polyneuropathy means that many nerves in different parts of the body are involved. Neuropathy can affect nerves that provide feeling (sensory neuropathy) or cause movement (motor neuropathy).

Symptoms affecting the nervous system reflect crown chakra tensions with father/authority, and the part of the body and function affected point to specific decisions the individual made in response to those tensions. With sensory neuropathy, the person has decided to not feel emotions in relation to the crown chakra tensions, and in the case of motor neuropathy, the individual has been paralyzing him/herself. See how the person experiences the symptom, and describe it from the point of view that they created it.

Polyp

A polyp is an abnormal growth of tissue projecting from a mucous membrane. As a growth, it represents something held in and not expressed. See the part of the body or the organ or function affected for further details about the inner cause.

Polyurea

Polyurea is excessive urination with abnormally large amounts of urine, reflecting insecurity and root chakra tensions about money, home and job. Because it is considered by some to be an early symptom of diabetes, it can reflect being angry with someone at home, but not feeling safe to express that anger. See Diabetes.

Polyuria

Polyuria is a medical term used to describe the symptom of increased frequency of urination. Anything affecting the elimination system reflects insecurity and tension in the root chakra parts of the person's life.

Post-nasal Drip

Rhinitis is a medical term for irritation and inflammation of the mucous membrane inside the nose. Common symptoms are a stuffy nose, runny nose and post-nasal drip. Because it is the nose that has been affected, the symptom is related to the root chakra, and the parts of the person's consciousness concerned with security (money, home, job), survival, trust and the person's sense of connection with their mother. The symptom points to insecurity or fear as a perceptual filter.

Post-Traumatic Stress Disorder (PTSD)

Post-traumatic stress disorder (PTSD) is an anxiety disorder caused by very stressful, frightening or distressing events. Tension is held in the root chakra, creating an intense emotional perceptual filter of fear.

Pott's Disease (Tuberculous Spondylitis)

Pott's disease is a partial destruction of the vertebral bones, caused by a tuberculous infection and often producing curvature of the spine, usually in the thorax. It reflects heart chakra tensions and anger with someone close, affecting the person's sense of stability, likely about tensions at home.

Pregnancy Disorders

Any pregnancy disorder or symptom having a tendency to affect a pregnancy reflects tension or ambivalence in the consciousness of the mother about having a child, considering the conditions in her life at that time.

Premenstrual Syndrome – See PMS

Primary Ciliary Dyskinesia (PCD)

This is a disorder that can affect the lungs, and is also known as immotile cilia syndrome and associated with Kartegener's syndrome. In people with PCD, the tiny hair-like structures (cilia) that are supposed to move mucus out of airways are abnormal or do not move. The mucus accumulates, causing blockage and infections. The lungs are associated with the heart chakra and the person's perceptions of love. The person doesn't feel the love around them, reflecting possible tension with someone close. This might also be due to a closed crown chakra, tensions or a lack of a sense of connection with the person's father, and therefore feeling isolated, as in a shell. Opening the shell and letting in the love from the father can prepare the way for the person feeling the love around them and allowing it in.

PCD can also affect the Fallopian tubes in women, and also the flagella of sperm in men, making it difficult to have children. If the person has difficulty feeling the love from their partner, it may affect their decision to have children. Also, because this is considered a genetic disorder, the person may feel unwilling to take a chance on passing along this symptom to children.

Primary Progressive Aphasia (PPA)

Primary progressive aphasia is caused by brain damage that affects language capabilities and thus a person's ability to communicate. It appears as a disorder of speaking, while comprehension remains relatively preserved. The person affected can understand, but doesn't communicate.

Because the brain is associated with the crown chakra, this symptom can reflect tensions with authority/father and the person holding themselves back from expressing themselves to authority, or it can reflect a sense of separation from someone close and holding oneself back from expressing or communicating about that.

Prolactinoma

Prolactinoma is a type of pituitary tumour (adenoma) affecting the production of prolactin, a hormone that triggers the breasts to produce milk. A common symptom is headache, pointing to crown chakra tensions and a sense of separation or isolation. Symptoms in women include milk flow from the breast in a woman who is not pregnant or nursing, breast tenderness, decreased sexual interest, infertility, stopping of menstruation not related to menopause or irregular menstruation, all pointing to tensions about having a child. It can seem like a 'false pregnancy', reflecting the woman's wish to be pregnant, though the infertility would reflect keeping herself from being pregnant – wanting to be pregnant but giving herself reasons to not have a child considering the circumstances in her life at that time.

In men it can include decreased sexual interest, enlargement of breast tissue, impotence and infertility, reflecting ambivalence about the male role and about being a father.

Symptoms caused by pressure from a larger tumour may include lethargy, runny nose and problems with the sense of smell, all pointing to root chakra tensions about money, home and job, and there may also be nausea and vomiting, pointing to solar plexus chakra anger or control issues, and vision changes; the person finding it difficult to look at circumstances in their life at that time.

Prolapse

In medicine, prolapse is a condition where organs fall down or slip out of place. It is used for organs protruding through the vagina or the rectum or for the misalignment of the valves of the heart. A spinal disc herniation is also sometimes called 'disc prolapse.' See Disc Herniation.

Rectal prolapse is a condition in which part of the wall or the entire wall of the rectum falls out of place. This reflects weakness in the root chakra – fear of losing something, or tension about holding on to something. It possibly reflects tensions at home.

Uterine prolapse (cystocele or pelvic organ prolapse) occurs when the female pelvic organs fall from their normal position, into or through the vagina. This reflects weakness in the root chakra, reflecting tensions at home. Because it can affect sexual activity, it points to tensions with a partner.

Prostate

The prostate gland is located at the level of the root chakra, which reflects something about trust, and it has a role in sexual intercourse. So when there are problems with the prostate gland, it reflects insecurity or mistrust in relation to a woman or women in general, either in relation to sex or in a more general sense.

Prostatitis

Prostatitis is a condition that involves inflammation of the prostate and sometimes the area around it. Because the prostate gland is located at the level of the root chakra, which reflects something about trust, it has a role in sexual intercourse and inflammation implies anger, prostatitis reflects anger and mistrust in relation to women, either in relation to sex or in a more general sense.

Pruritis Ani

Pruritus ani is a persistent itch or irritation around the anus. Because of the location at the level of the root chakra, which also is associated with the elimination system, this symptom implies irritation about an unsatisfactory situation at home, or in relation to money.

Psoriasis

Psoriasis is a skin disease that causes itchy or sore patches of thick, red skin with silvery scales. It usually appears on the elbows, knees, scalp, back, face, palms and feet, but it can show up on other parts of the body. It is considered to be related to problems with the immune system, associated with the heart chakra, and therefore having something to do with the area of relationships and the person's perceptions of love.

As a skin problem, it represents sensitivity in the area of the solar plexus chakra, a perceived threat to one's sense of personal power to be oneself, though to further understand the inner cause, see the part of the body affected and the possible effect of the symptom. For example, if it affects the scalp it is solar plexus energy, or feeling nervous or threatened, in relation to the crown chakra, and the relationship with father/ authority.

On the face, it would reflect sensitivity about letting people close, being nervous about what others might see in the person.

On the elbows and palms it would represent nervousness about going for and accepting the fulfilment of one's goals, and on the knees and feet it would represent sensitivity about solar plexus energy in the area of the root chakra – in relation to money, home and job. If it affects much of the body, it can be understood that the person is uncomfortable in terms of intimate contact – so it can represent issues of freedom, power or control affecting the person in the area of intimate contact.

Psoriatic Arthritis (Psoriatic Arthropathy)

Psoriatic arthritis (also arthritis psoriatica, arthropathic psoriasis or psoriatic arthropathy) is a type of inflammatory arthritis that can develop in people who have the chronic skin condition psoriasis. Common symptoms include sausage-like swelling in the fingers or toes, known as dactylitis, as well as pain, swelling or stiffness in one or more joints, joints that are red or warm to the touch, pain in and around the feet and ankles, especially inflammation in the Achilles tendon or in the sole of the foot, pain in the area of the sacrum (the lower back, above the tailbone) and extreme exhaustion that does not go away with adequate rest. All of this points to tensions in the root chakra, and therefore in the parts of the person's consciousness having to do with security, survival and trust, and the parts of the person's life that represent security – money, home, job. When the fingers are affected, there is insecurity about the person accepting the fulfilment of their goals; insecurity about having what they really want, most likely about the root chakra parts of their life.

Psychosis

When a person suffers from psychosis they are not able to tell the difference between reality and what is in their imagination; it is a loss of contact with reality in a way that affects their ability to function and interact. The major symptoms, aside from delusions and hallucinations, are disorganized speech and behaviour, lack of emotional expression and apathy. They feel isolated in an alternative reality in which they do not feel understood, reflecting tensions in the brow and crown chakras.

It should be mentioned that there is a possibility to function in alternative realities such as healing while remaining functional in what is considered society's 'norm', though that might be uncomfortable if the person is surrounded by others who judge those alternative realities, resulting in the person closing their crown chakra, creating in them a sense of isolation because of a pejorative label imposed on them because of their non-ordinary experiences and perceptions.

Psychosomatic Problems

Psychosomatic means mind (psyche) and body (soma). A psychosomatic disorder is a disease that involves both mind and body. The term 'psycho-somatic disorder' is mainly used to mean 'a physical disease that is thought to be caused, or made worse, by mental or emotional factors.' This book you are reading now is based on the idea that all symptoms begin with something happening in the consciousness, regardless of the apparent 'physical' cause or trigger. Thus, all symptoms are psychosomatic, and it is therefore possible in principle to release them when the inner conditions change. See the specific symptom to understand the tension in the consciousness associated with it.

Ptosis

Ptosis is a drooping or falling of the upper eyelid, possibly affecting vision in that eye. If it is the male eye affected (right eye in a right-handed person) it reflects tension with or about a male, with men or a man in their life at that time; and if it affects the female eye, tension with or about a female in their life at that time. If the right/left polarity is described as will/emotions, it could represent the person not seeing what they really want, or not seeing what they really feel. See Eyelids, Eyes.

Pubic Bone Pain (Symphysis Pubis Dysfunction – SPD)

During pregnancy or birth, about one in thirty-five women will experience intense pubic bone pain (pelvic pain) and may find it difficult to walk, climb stairs and perform other movements and activities (including sex) that involve the pelvic bones. This pain is a result of separation of the symphysis pubis, which is a joint in the very front part of the pelvic bone structure. The location points to tensions in the root chakra (insecurity) in relation to the process of pregnancy or birth, and/or in relation to having sex during pregnancy or shortly afterwards.

Pulmonary Disease/Lung Disease

Any pulmonary disease affects the lungs and therefore breathing. The lungs and the element of air are related to the heart chakra, and any symptom that affects breathing is related to tensions with someone close.

The person's relationship with air reflects their relationship with love, in terms of letting it in (breathing in) or expressing it (breathing out). See Lungs.

Pulmonary Embolism

A pulmonary embolism is a blood clot in the artery bringing blood and therefore nourishment to the lung. It reflects heart chakra tension with someone close, and difficulty letting in the love from that person, not allowing oneself to be nourished by the love.

Pulmonary Emphysema – See Emphysema

Pyelonephritis

Pyelonephritis is an inflammation of both the lining of the pelvis and the kidney. The symptoms are pain and tenderness in the part of the back between the ribs and the hip, with fever, and usually with frequent, urgent and/or painful urination. Nausea and vomiting are common. The parts of the body affected are related to the root chakra, and the symptoms therefore reflect tensions there, experienced as insecurity, and a sense of helplessness about something happening in the person's life that they feel unhappy with though powerless to do anything about. This perceived lack of power is also reflected in the vomiting and nausea, tensions in the solar plexus chakra and a sense of things going out of control. The fever reflects anger.

Pyorrhoea

Pyorrhoea, or periodontitis, is an advanced stage of periodontal disease in which the ligaments and bones that support the teeth become inflamed and infected with pus. The teeth and gums are related to the root chakra. Inflammation implies anger – thus, this symptom represents anger or tensions in the root chakra parts of the person's life, and therefore the parts of the person's consciousness dealing with security and those things that represent security – money, home, job.

Pyrosis – See Heartburn

Quinsy – See Peritonsillar Abscess

Rabies

Rabies affects the brain, where it causes swelling or inflammation. This reflects crown chakra tensions with father/authority. Symptoms may include convulsions and loss of muscle function, and since these are associated with the solar plexus chakra, it can relate to solar plexus tensions in relation to authority, a perceived lack of power in relation to authority. Difficulty swallowing reflects difficulty 'swallowing' or accepting some situation in the person's life at the time the symptom began.

Rachitis – See Rickets

Rash

A rash is a change in the skin caused by an irritation that can result from an allergy, infection or skin problem like eczema or psoriasis. It is solar plexus energy representing anger, and the part of the body affected reflects the source or effect of the anger.

Raynaud's Disease/Phenomenon

Raynaud's phenomenon (RP) is a condition resulting in a particular series of discolorations of the fingers and/or the toes after exposure to changes in temperature (cold or hot) or emotional events. During an attack of Raynaud's, affected areas of the skin usually turn white at first. Then they often turn blue, feel cold and numb, and the sense of touch is dulled. As circulation improves, the affected areas may turn red, throb, tingle or swell. In terms of the response to the emotional event at the time the condition began, the symptoms of difficulty in circulating blood to the fingers and toes point to the circulation of love (blood, heart chakra) at home (feet, root chakra) and the individual's beliefs about having what they want and what will make them happy (hands), most likely in terms of their perceptions of love. Numbness can be described as keeping oneself from feeling, avoiding going into the emotions of what is happening in one's life, related to the area affected and the chakra associated with that part or function.

Rectum

The rectum is the final or terminal segment of the digestive system in which faeces accumulate just prior to discharge. The rectum is continuous with the sigmoid colon and extends thirteen to fifteen cm (five to six inches) to the anus. It is related to the root chakra, and any symptom involving the rectum therefore reflects root chakra tensions about security, survival, trust and those parts of the person's life related to security – money, home, job, mother.

Recurrent Respiratory Papillomatosis (RRP) – See Human Papillomavirus (HPV)

Reflux – See Acid Reflux

Regurgitation – See Vomit

Reproductive System

Any symptom affecting the reproductive system could result in an inability to have children, thus reflecting the person's ambivalence about having a child at the time the symptom began, because of conditions in their life at that time.

Respiratory System

The respiratory system is made up of the organs in the body that help the person to breathe. It includes the airways, lungs and the respiratory muscles. Because it is associated with the heart chakra and the element of air, symptoms affecting the respiratory system therefore reflect tensions with someone close to the person's heart (a partner, parent, sibling or child) and difficulty letting in the love from that person.

Restless Legs Syndrome (RLS)

Restless legs syndrome (RLS) is a neurological disorder characterized by an irresistible urge to move one's body to stop uncomfortable or odd sensations. It most commonly affects the legs, but can affect the arms, torso, head and even phantom limbs. Moving the affected body part provides temporary relief. As a neurological disorder, it reflects tensions with father/authority, or a sense of isolation or separation from someone close. The part of the body affected points to specific tensions. Thus, when the legs are affected it reflects root chakra tensions and insecurity affecting the will or the emotions, the torso reflects heart chakra tensions with someone close and the arms reflect the person talking him/herself out of going for their goals.

Retention of Water – See Oedema

Retinal Separation, Retinal Detachment

Retinal detachment refers to the movement of the retina away from the inner wall of the eyeball, resulting in a sudden defect in vision. If it is the male eye (right eye in right-handed people), it points to a sense of separation from a male at the time the symptom began. If it is the female eye that is affected, it reflects a sense of separation from a female.

Retinitis Pigmentosa

Retinitis pigmentosa is a condition in which there is dystrophy or damage to the photoreceptors of the retina and of the pigment epithelium underneath the photoreceptors, due to pigmentation that begins and settles within the layers of the neural retina. The effect is increasing tunnel vision. Pigment is associated with the crown chakra, and is therefore to do with authority/father or a sense of separation or isolation, which would be the eventual effect of the symptom as its logical conclusion is blindness.

The symptom therefore points to a sense of separation or isolation, or tensions with authority, at the time the symptom began, increasing as the symptom progresses. If it affects just one eye, the male eye (right eye in those born right-handed), it points to not seeing the male or separation from a male in the person's life, and the emotional eye points to separation from a female at the time the symptom began.

Rett's Syndrome

Rett's syndrome is a neurodevelopmental disorder of the grey matter of the brain that almost exclusively affects female children but has also been found in male patients. It reflects a closed crown chakra and a reaction to a perceived lack of contact with the person's father. An abnormally small head and poor head growth may be evident. Difficulties walking, scoliosis and gastrointestinal difficulties point to root chakra tensions as well, and a possible perceived lack of contact with the mother. Screaming fits and inconsolable crying reflect the child's frustration at the sense of isolation. Breathing difficulties reflect heart chakra tensions and not feeling the contact with the parents and therefore not feeling the love, and developmental difficulties reflect a wish to return to an earlier infant state when there may have been more of a sense of contact with the parents.

Rheumatism

Rheumatism (or rheumatic disorder) is a non-specific term for medical conditions that affect connective tissue and the joints, which are associated with the root chakra. The effect is immobilization of the affected part(s). The condition points to the person immobilizing him or herself because of insecurity. See specific parts of the body affected for further details about how or why the person has been immobilizing him or herself.

Rheumatoid Arthritis

Rheumatoid arthritis is described as an autoimmune disease that results in a chronic, systemic inflammatory disorder that may affect many tissues and organs, but principally attacks flexible joints. Because the immune system is associated with the heart chakra and the area of relationships, and the joints are associated with the root chakra, the symptom reflects the person immobilizing themselves because of insecurity, possibly about tensions in their relationship with someone close.

Rhinitis

Rhinitis is a medical term for irritation and inflammation of the mucous membrane inside the nose. Common symptoms are a stuffy nose, runny nose and post-nasal drip. The nose is related to the root chakra, so insecurity, tensions at home and the relationship with the mother, and because it involves taking in air through the nose, and air is the element related to the heart chakra and perceptions of love, it can be related to difficulty letting in love from the mother, or difficulty letting in the love at home.

Allergic rhinitis may cause additional symptoms, such as sneezing and nasal itching, coughing (to do with the heart chakra, pushing away the love, the person being angry at someone close to their heart), headache (crown chakra tensions, sense of separation/isolation), fatigue (root chakra tensions) and cognitive impairment; not thinking clearly. The allergens may also affect the eyes, causing watery, reddened or itchy eyes and puffiness around the eyes – looking like the person is crying and finding it difficult to look at something happening in their life.

Ribs

Symptoms affecting the ribs reflect tensions in the heart and/or solar plexus chakras, depending on which ribs are affected and which chakra is closest, and whether they are on the will side (right side in right-handed people) or the emotional side, reflecting a reaction of something happening contrary to what the person wants, or an emotional reaction to events at that time. Heart chakra tensions reflect conflict with someone close, and solar plexus tensions reflect reactions involving power, control or freedom.

Rickets

Rickets is a disorder caused by a lack of vitamin D, calcium or phosphate. It leads to softening and weakening of the bones. The skeletal system is associated with the root chakra, and therefore to the parts of the person's consciousness associated with security (home) and the person's sense of connection with their mother. This could be a reaction to tensions in the consciousness of the mother about her capability to raise the child, or if there is a sense of separation from the father at that time, a closed crown chakra that effectively creates a sense of isolation for the child, even separating them from feeling their connection with their mother.

Right Side of Body

In right-handed people, the right side of the body is considered the will side, or the male side. For people born left-handed, the right side of their body is considered the emotional side, or the female side. These descriptors are useful in identifying the inner cause to symptoms. When symptoms typically affect primarily one side of the body, see whether it is the male side or the female side, and identify that with the person's relationship with their father and their mother. Also understand that there may be difficulty with the male side and female side of the brain communicating with each other, reflecting the person's reaction to a lack of communication between his/her mother and father.

Ringing in the Ears – See Tinnitus

Ringworm

Ringworm (tinea) is caused by a fungal infection on the skin. It often makes a pattern in the shape of a ring, but not always. Sometimes it is just a red, itchy rash. A fungal infection reflects something 'eating away' in the person's consciousness, a background irritation that has come to the surface. See the part of the body affected to understand what the irritation is about.

One form of the symptom may be Jock itch, a rash in the skin folds of the groin, pointing to root chakra tensions and insecurity. It may also spread to the inner thighs or buttocks. This may reflect insecurity about sexuality or sensitivities about being naked in front of others. Because it is considered contagious, it implies a sense of separation or isolation because of the insecurity.

Ringworm of the hand looks like athlete's foot. The skin on the palm of the hand gets thick, dry and scaly, and skin between the fingers may be moist and have open sores. Symptoms affecting the hands reflect difficulty accepting the fulfilment of one's goals, and because the symptom is considered contagious, the symptom reflects the person avoiding contact with others.

Roger's Disease

Roger's disease is a defect in the septum that separates the ventricles of the heart. It reflects heart chakra tensions and therefore difficulties with the person's perceptions of love. When detected in infants or children, it can be a reaction to a perceived lack of contact with one or both parents.

Root Canal Problems

The 'root canal' is the term used to describe the natural cavity within the centre of the tooth. The pulp or pulp chamber is the soft area within the root canal. The tooth's nerve lies within the root canal. A tooth's nerve and pulp can become irritated, inflamed and infected. The teeth are related to the root chakra, and the parts of the person's consciousness related to security, survival and trust; and the parts of their life associated with security – money, home, job and mother. The jaw, as it holds the teeth, is associated with the solar plexus. Thus, this symptom can be associated with tensions in the root chakra parts of the person's life, and possible anger or irritation in these areas.

Root Chakra Tensions

The root chakra is associated with the parts of the consciousness related to security, survival and trust, and the parts of the person's life related to security – money, home, job and mother. The person's relationship with their mother sets a pattern for their relationship with everything related to security – money, home, and job. Root chakra tensions that can be correlated with physical and emotional symptoms include a sense of separation from the person's mother, tension or anger with their mother or not seeing their mother as a nourishing energy.

In terms of money, the tension may reflect worry about debt or not having enough money, not feeling nourished on their job in terms of being sufficiently paid for what they do or not having a sense of satisfaction with their job, or tensions in the job environment.

In terms of home, the tensions could be about the physical home and its location, or the home environment (harmony in the home and family environment); not feeling safe at home.

Tensions on the male side of the root chakra (right side in someone right-handed) can represent insecurity with a male or not feeling nourished by a male, and tensions on the female side of the root chakra can represent insecurity with a female or not feeling nourished by a female. If the right/left polarity is described as will/emotions, tensions on the will side would reflect insecurity or a person's lack of trust in his/her will, not trusting themselves to do what they want; and on the emotional side, emotional insecurity, not standing on their own with regard to their emotions.

Rosacea

Rosacea is a skin disease that causes redness and pimples on the nose, cheeks, chin and forehead. It reflects solar plexus tension, anger and a sense of embarrassment or shame, since there may be a feeling of not wanting to be visible, wanting to hide one's face.

Roseola

Roseola is a mild infection that affects babies and young children. It generally causes three days of high fever (often over 103 degrees F); this then subsides and the child breaks out in a flat or bumpy red rash, usually starting around the neck, back and chest, then spreading out. It can last from a few days to a couple of weeks. Fever and rash point to anger or frustration with the parents about something that happened when the symptom began.

Round Shoulders

Round shoulders is a postural defect in which the shoulders are drawn forward, the head is extended and the chin pokes forward. While the neck and shoulders are associated with the throat chakra, the effect of this symptom is to protect a sensitive heart chakra, reflecting sensitivities in the area of relationships; sensitivity about feeling loved.

Rubella (German Measles)

Rubella (also known as German measles) is a viral infection that used to be common in children. The patient develops a rash that typically starts around the ears, from where it spreads all over the body in tiny pink spots. It reflects anger. Up to one week before the rash appears, the patient can suffer a light cold, consisting of a cough and sore throat and/or swelling in the neck and base of the skull (due to the enlargement of the lymph nodes), again pointing to anger about something at home.

Sore red eyes (conjunctivitis) can occur and make the person look like they are upset or crying about something, and there can be joint pains, primarily affecting adults, reflecting root chakra tensions about a situation at home. Brain inflammation may also occur, reflecting crown chakra tensions and anger with father/authority.

Rubeola – See Measles

Sacral Chakra Tensions

Sacral chakra tensions that can result in symptoms include tensions about food, sex or having children, or a strong emotional shock that the person has had difficulty dealing with that can affect them in these areas. In terms of food, it may be a food addiction, a compulsive need for a particular food, though this is generally related to the symptom associated with the effects of having that food. Tensions can be about inner conflict and not listening to one's appetite, but rather trusting an external 'authority' about what one should eat.

In the area of sexuality, tensions can include inhibitions and tension about what the body is attracted to and conditions the individual finds interesting sexually, and suppressing these responses of their body, rather than acknowledging them and then deciding whether or not to act on them. Ambivalence about having children is related to this chakra as well.

SAD – See Seasonal Affective Disorder

Saddle Back – See Lordosis

Salivary Glands

The salivary glands produce saliva, which is important to lubricate your mouth, help with swallowing, protect your teeth against bacteria and aid in the digestion of food. When there is a problem with the salivary glands or ducts, symptoms may include swelling, dry mouth, pain, fever and foul-tasting drainage into the mouth, affecting not only eating but expressing oneself and allowing others to get close, reflecting throat chakra tensions and unexpressed anger.

Salpingitis

Salpingitis is an infection and inflammation in the Fallopian tubes that can result in infertility. Symptoms of chronic salpingitis may also include recurring severe period pain, painful intercourse, vaginal discharge and poor general health, reflecting the person giving herself reasons to not have children, likely because of anger with a sexual partner.

Sarcoma

A sarcoma is a type of cancer that develops from certain tissues, like bone or muscle. The main types of sarcoma are: osteosarcoma, which develops from bone, and soft tissue sarcomas, which can develop from soft tissues like fat, muscle, nerves, fibrous tissues, blood vessels or deep skin tissues. Thus, malignant tumours made of cancerous bone, cartilage, fat, muscle or blood vessel tissues are, by definition, considered sarcomas.

Cancer represents something held in and not expressed, and the part of the body affected shows what this was. Cancerous bone points to root chakra tensions, muscle sarcomas point to issues of power, blood vessel sarcomas point to heart chakra tensions with someone close, in terms of what was happening in the person's life at the time the symptom began.

Regardless of the part of the body affected, see the eventual possible logical conclusion of the symptom – death – from the point of view that everything begins in the consciousness to understand that the person has decided that the situation they are in is unacceptable, and they would rather die than continue with that situation in their life. They must resolve this tension in order to have something to look forward to, something to live for.

SARS (Severe Acute Respiratory Syndrome)

Severe acute respiratory syndrome (SARS) is a viral respiratory illness. Initial symptoms are flu-like and may include fever, muscle pain, lethargy, cough and sore throat, pointing to unexpressed anger with someone close and a feeling of powerlessness in the situation. Shortness of breath may occur later, pointing to difficulty letting in the love. Because the symptom seems specific to a particular region or part of the world, it can point to group consciousness tensions that the individual has accepted.

Scabies

Scabies is an infestation of the skin by the human itch mite. The microscopic scabies mite burrows into the upper layer of the skin, where it lives and lays its eggs. The most common symptoms of scabies are intense itching and a pimple-like skin rash. The superficial burrows of scabies usually occur in the areas of the hands, feet, wrists, elbows, back, buttocks and external genitals. The symptom points to something 'eating away' in the person's consciousness, something bothering them in the background of their consciousness, and the part of the body affected reflects what the sensitivity is about. For example, if the genitals are affected, it points to tensions in the area of sexuality. Because the symptom is considered contagious, see how the person has been isolating him/herself with crown chakra tensions with father/authority or a sense of separation from someone close.

Scalp

The scalp is associated with the crown chakra, and therefore with the parts of the person's consciousness concerned with father/authority, and feeling connected or separate. When there are symptoms affecting the scalp, they are reflecting tensions in these areas. Skin problems affecting the scalp point to solar plexus tensions (power, control, anger) in relation to father/authority, or causing a sense of separation from someone.

Scapula (Shoulder Blade)

The scapula is the large, flat, triangular bone forming the back part of the shoulder. Symptoms affecting this bone or in the area of this bone reflect heart chakra tensions with someone close, and when shoulder or arm movement is affected, reflect keeping oneself from setting and going for goals in terms of what one wants or what will make one happy in the area of relationships.

Scarlet Fever

Scarlet fever is a bacterial illness that causes a distinctive pink-red rash that feels like sandpaper to touch and may spread to the ears, neck and chest. The rash may be itchy. Other symptoms include a high temperature, a flushed face and a red, swollen tongue. These symptoms point to anger, possibly unexpressed, with someone close.

Schamberg's Disease

Schamberg's disease, or progressive pigmented purpuric dermatitis, is a purplish discoloration of the skin that usually affects the legs and is caused by blood leaking from small vessels near the skin's surface. When the legs are affected, it points to tensions in the root chakra, and therefore the parts of the person's consciousness concerned with security, survival and trust; and the parts of their life dealing with security – money, home, job, mother. Because it involves the blood vessels in the legs, it points to circulation of love with the mother, and because it is also associated with itching, it can reflect a sense of irritation with the mother or with root chakra issues – money, home and job.

Scheuermann's Disease – See Kyphosis

Schizophrenia

Schizophrenia is defined by Western traditions as a mental health condition that includes a range of different psychological symptoms, including hallucinations (hearing or seeing things that 'do not exist'), delusions (unusual beliefs not based on reality 'that often contradict the evidence') muddled thoughts based on the 'hallucinations' or 'delusions' and certain changes in behaviour. Doctors often describe schizophrenia as a psychotic illness. This can mean for them that sometimes a person may not be able to distinguish their own thoughts and ideas from reality.

It should be pointed out that by this definition, certain valid though non-ordinary states of consciousness and spiritual experiences are classified in the West as schizophrenia, and the only problem may be the pejorative label, making the person feel that they have something wrong with them. Of course, in these cases, the person should be able to remain functional in society and in their everyday life. Spiritual healing may be considered a 'positive psychosis'.

A hallucination is when a person experiences a sensation but there is nothing or nobody there in the physical plane to account for it. A 'hallucination' can involve any of the senses, but the most common is hearing voices. It should be considered that the person might be experiencing clairvoyance, clairaudience, channelling, etc., as the result of an opening of their brow chakra, the 'third eye.'

A delusion is a belief held with complete conviction, even though it is considered by others to be based on a mistaken, strange or 'unrealistic' view. Again, certain valid spiritual experiences and healing perceptions could be described in this way.

Someone experiencing a paranoid delusion may believe they are being harassed or persecuted. They may think they are being chased, followed, watched, plotted against or poisoned, often by a family member or friend. This could be seen as the effect of a closed root chakra, resulting in insecurity or fear as a perceptual filter, possibly combined with a closed crown chakra, resulting in a sense of isolation.

Some people who experience delusions find different meanings in everyday events or occurrences. They may believe people on TV or in newspaper articles are communicating messages to them alone, or that there are hidden messages in the colours of cars passing in the street. This can also be understood, though, as the person experiencing a sense of connection with and communication from their spirit, their higher self.

People experiencing psychosis often have trouble keeping track of their thoughts and conversations. Some people find it hard to concentrate and will drift from one idea to another. This reflects a closed root chakra and not being grounded.

Some people may describe their thoughts as being controlled by someone else, or say that their thoughts are not their own or that thoughts have been planted in their mind by someone else. This can also be understood as a sense of empathy, a connection at the level of the crown chakra, experiencing another person's experience, a not uncommon state for some healers. A lack of understanding of these valid though non-ordinary states of consciousness can result in insecurity and thus tension in the root chakra.

Another recognized feeling is that thoughts are disappearing, as though someone is removing them from their mind. Some people feel their body is being taken over and someone else is directing their movements and actions. Those functioning as spiritual 'channels' do this consciously, allowing themselves to be 'used' by spirits not on the physical plane.

Multiple personalities can be created as a way to allow a freedom of expression as a reaction to a closed crown chakra and thus tensions with a controlling authority.

Sciatica

Sciatica is the name given to any sort of pain that is caused by irritation or compression of the sciatic nerve that runs from the lumbar area down the legs. Because the pain begins at the level of the sacral chakra, it represents tension about food, sex or having children, affecting or affected by questions of trust in a man (male leg) or a woman (female leg), lack of trust in the will (will leg) or having a sense of emotional insecurity (emotional leg); not standing on one's own two feet with regard to their emotions. If the eventual effect of the symptom could be inability to walk, it reflects the person giving themselves reasons to stay in an unhappy situation, keeping themselves from walking away.

Scleroderma

Scleroderma is a group of diseases that cause abnormal growth of connective tissue, the material inside your body that gives your tissues their shape and helps keep them strong. In scleroderma, the tissue gets hard or thick. It can cause swelling or pain in the muscles and joints, and in that case would be associated with root chakra tensions and solar plexus tensions, and the person immobilizing him/herself through insecurity and a perceived lack of power.

The part(s) of the body affected reflect more precisely the inner cause, depending on the function affected. If the oesophagus is affected, for example, it can represent the person having difficulty accepting or 'swallowing' a situation in their life at the time the symptom began or was discovered. Red spots on the face can reflect a sense of embarrassment, with the person feeling they need to hide their face.

Scoliosis (Curvature of the Spine)

Anything affecting the entire spinal column is related to the root chakra, and therefore issues of insecurity, not feeling safe at home or not experiencing the mother as a source of nourishment and security. In this case, however, there is a curvature at specific locations that can be related to the chakras. See which chakras are involved, those closest to the curvature and whether the tensions are located on the will side or the emotional side. Thus, for a right-handed person, if the curve at the level of the solar plexus is toward the emotional side, this reflects emotional tensions about power, control and/or freedom; and if on the will side, tension in the person's will about these issues.

If there is also curvature at the level of the heart chakra, see which side has the tension and understand it as representing tensions about the combination – something to do with solar plexus issues in the area of relationships or tensions about personal freedom when in a relationship.

As always, see when the symptom began, and also when the symptom was diagnosed and what was happening in the person's life at that time.

Scotopic Sensitivity Syndrome – See Meares–Irlen Syndrome

Scurvy

Scurvy is a disease that occurs when there is a severe lack of vitamin C (ascorbic acid) in the diet. It causes general weakness, anaemia, gum disease and a rash on the legs, reflecting root chakra tensions and insecurity about money, home, job and mother.

Seasickness – See Motion Sickness

Seasonal Affective Disorder (SAD)

Seasonal affective disorder or SAD, also known as winter depression, winter blues, summer depression, summer blues or seasonal depression, is a disorder in which people who have normal mental health throughout most of the year experience depressive symptoms in the winter or summer. Depression is a sense of powerlessness to do something about an unhappy situation, and can then be related to the situation the person is unhappy about during the season in which they feel affected.

Seizures

Seizures happen because of sudden, abnormal electrical activity in the brain, which is associated with the crown chakra. Thus, there is tension about father/authority, or a sense of separation from someone. Often the symptom is triggered by fear, and the person goes out of their body, pointing to root chakra tensions about money, home, job or mother. It can also reflect the person reacting to possible separation or tension between their parents, something happening with the father that results in a sense of separation from the mother.

Senile Dementia, Senility

Senility refers to mental deterioration and infirmity that is often associated with old age, as in severe memory problems. It is related to root chakra tensions and insecurity or fear, possibly about mortality and the apparent inevitability of death, these tensions manifesting as not being present with what is happening around them. There may also be crown chakra considerations; feeling isolated or separated from others due to society's attitudes toward aging.

Sepsis/Septicaemia

Septicaemia, formerly called blood poisoning, is an infection resulting from the presence of bacteria in the blood. It often begins with a high fever, chills, weakness and excessive sweating, followed by a decrease in blood pressure. It can arise from infections throughout the body, including in the lungs, abdomen or urinary tract, reflecting tensions in the heart chakra (tensions and anger with someone close to the person's heart, perceptions of love) and root chakra (tensions at home). Symptoms of confusion and decreased urine output also point to root chakra tensions (security, survival, trust).

Severe Myoclonic Epilepsy of Infancy (SMEI) – See Dravet Syndrome

Sexual Dysfunction

Sexual dysfunction refers to a difficulty experienced by an individual or a couple during any stage of a normal sexual activity, including desire, preference, arousal or orgasm. It can include erectile dysfunction (ED) and premature or delayed ejaculation in men, spasms of the vagina, pain with sexual intercourse and problems with sexual desire (libido) and response. From the point of view that we each create our reality, the person affected has been keeping him/herself from having sex, and reasons for that may be tensions with his/her partner, in which case the attention held in the solar plexus chakra (anger, conflict) can prevent the attention going to the sacral chakra. Other possibilities are root chakra tensions (insecurity, lack of trust) or societal values that may be in conflict with the person's sexual appetite.

Sexually Transmitted Disease

Any sexually transmitted disease, even those that do not affect the sexual organs, reflect ambivalence about sexuality, and possibly conflict around sexual values based on what the individual may perceive in others. The person may feel that their own sexual values are 'wrong'.

Shingles

Herpes zoster (or simply zoster), commonly called shingles and also known as zona, is a viral disease characterized by a painful skin rash with blisters in a limited area on one side of the body, often in a stripe. It is associated with the varicella zoster virus, which affects the nerves. Because the nerves are involved, there is an association with the crown chakra, which controls the brain and the nervous system, and because it causes blisters, it is associated with anger. Thus, shingles is associated with anger that creates a sense of separation from someone, and the part of the body affected and the chakra associated with that part of the body reflect further details.

For example, if it is one side of the neck, it is associated with not expressing what one wants or feels (depending on whether the will side or the emotional side is affected), and if the skin is affected on one side of the body at the level of the heart chakra, we can see how that reflects the specific tension in the consciousness in the area of relationships.

Shins

The shinbone is the larger of the two bones in the leg below the knee, and it is therefore associated with the root chakra and with the parts of the consciousness concerned with security and trust. A symptom involving this part represents a shock, stimulating tension or a violation of trust on the will side (right side in right-handed people) or, on the emotional side, reflecting issues of trust with a male or a female.

Shoulders

The shoulders are associated with the throat chakra and therefore expression. Tension in the shoulders can represent something not expressed or not communicated. Since the throat chakra also controls the arms and hands, a symptom involving the shoulder can result in immobility of the arms, which represent going for one's goals. The person affected can thus be said to be talking themselves out of going for their goals, talking to themselves in a way that discourages them from going for a specific goal concerning what they want (on the will side) or for what makes them happy (emotional side). A sense of heaviness on the shoulders can be experienced as carrying a heavy burden, a sense of responsibility that the person perceives as keeping them from going for their goals.

Shoulder Blade – See Scapula

Sickle Cell Anaemia (Sickle Cell Disease)

Sickle cell disease changes normal, round red blood cells into cells shaped like crescent moons or sickles. Normal red blood cells move easily through the blood vessels, taking oxygen to every part of the body, but sickled cells can get stuck and block blood vessels, which stops the oxygen from getting through. That can cause a lot of pain and can also harm organs, muscles and bones. The blood circulatory system is associated with the heart chakra and with the person's perceptions of love. The person is not allowing him/herself to be nourished by the love around them. See the specific organ, muscle or bone affected for further details of decisions made by the person affected.

Silicosis

Silicosis is a lung disease caused by inhaling tiny bits of silica. Symptoms can include shortness of breath, cough, bluish skin, fever, chest pains, loss of appetite and fatigue, reflecting heart chakra tensions and anger with someone close, as well as root chakra tensions at home.

Sinusitis

Sinusitis is inflammation of the air cavities within the passages of the nose. Inflammation implies anger, and the nose is associated with the root chakra and therefore the parts of the consciousness concerned with security, survival and trust; and the parts of the person's life associated with security – money, home, job, mother. Thus, sinusitis is related to anger about the root chakra parts of the person's consciousness at the time the symptom began. Symptoms can include sinus headache or pressure or pain in the sinuses, pointing to brow chakra tensions, or the person feeling not seen for who they are behind the role; facial tenderness, as if they had felt slapped in the face; fever, implying anger; feeling of nasal stuffiness, difficulty taking in the air, difficulty letting in the love at home or from the mother; sore throat, reflecting unexpressed anger; and cough, signalling heart chakra tensions, pushing away someone close to their heart and anger with someone close.

Sjogren's Syndrome

The main symptoms of Sjogren's syndrome are dry mouth and dry eyes. The person has been unhappy about something but keeping themselves from crying, and has had difficulty communicating with someone. Because Sjogren's syndrome is described as an autoimmune condition, it points to tensions with someone close to the person's heart. In women (who are most commonly affected), the glands responsible for keeping the vagina moist can also be affected, leading to vaginal dryness and therefore resistance to sexual contact, again pointing to possible tensions with someone close.

Skeleton

The skeleton as a whole is associated with the root chakra, and therefore with the parts of the person's consciousness related to security, survival, trust and their connection with their mother. Systemic symptoms (osteoporosis, systemic arthritis) that affect the entire skeleton would thus point to root chakra tensions, though difficulties in a particular part of the skeleton, such as a broken bone, would reflect tension in the chakra associated with that part of the body, possibly pointing also to insecurity about that function. Thus, a broken right arm would reflect tension in the throat chakra concerning the person 'reaching' for what they want, possibly because of insecurity about going for that goal.

Skin, General

In general, the skin is associated with the solar plexus chakra and therefore issues of power, control, freedom and self-definition. If the skin in general is affected (for example eczema over much of the body) it could represent issues of nervousness about being oneself, and how one appears to others, though the possible logical consequence of the symptom (sensitivity about intimate contact) could also reflect issues of personal freedom affecting the person in the area of intimate contact.

Skin symptoms in a particular part of the body reflect solar plexus energy affecting that part; thus, skin conditions over the area of the heart could represent solar plexus energy (control issues, anger, conflict) in the area of relationships.

Skin Cancer

The skin is associated with the solar plexus chakra and one's appearance to others, the face one shows the world. Cancer represents something held in and not expressed, as a reaction to some strong condition in one's life at the time the symptom began or was discovered. Thus, the skin cancer represents tension about how one appears to others within the context of the difficult situation in the person's life at the time the symptom began, serious enough for the person to decide they may prefer to die rather than face life with that situation.

Sleep Apnoea – See Apnoea

Slipped Disc

A slipped disc, also known as a prolapsed or herniated disc, is where one of the discs in the spine ruptures and the gel inside leaks out. This can cause back pain as well as pain in other areas of the body. The location of the disc and the chakra associated with that location, and the part of the body affected and its associated chakra, as well as the function affected, would point to the specific tensions in the consciousness.

Smallpox

Smallpox gets its name from its most common symptom: small blisters erupting on the face, arms and body that become pustules (filled with pus). Symptoms of smallpox include flu-like fatigue, headache, body ache and occasionally vomiting, high fever, mouth sores and blisters that spread the virus into the throat. These point to tensions in the root chakra and crown chakra, insecurity and a sense of isolation, anger, frustration and a sense of helplessness to change difficult conditions in the person's life. Smallpox is considered to have been eradicated in the world and to no longer exist as a risk.

Smoking Addiction – See Addiction

Sneezing

Sneezing is generally considered a normal body reaction designed to clear the nose. The nose is associated with the root chakra. Thus, sneezing reflects a clearing of the root chakra, allowing the person to breathe freely through the nose, reflecting trust in allowing in the love. Excessive sneezing can be related to throat chakra irritation combined with root chakra sensitivities – insecurity about expressing anger – or anger about the root chakra parts of the person's life – mother, money, home or job.

Snoring

Snoring is the vibration of sound due to blocked air movement during breathing while sleeping. Because air is associated with the heart chakra, the person's relationship with air reflects their relationship with love. Difficulty letting in the air thus reflects difficulty letting in the love, possibly in relation to root chakra considerations with home or the person's mother. Because it discourages contact with a bed partner, it reflects resistance to close heart chakra connections.

Solar Plexus

The solar plexus is associated with the solar plexus chakra, and therefore with considerations of power, control and freedom. It is also associated with the mental body, and tension here can be related to excessive mental activity and control issues. Tension in this area can also reflect anger.

Solar Plexus Chakra Tensions

The solar plexus chakra is associated with the parts of the person's consciousness related to power, control and freedom, as well as self-definition. Solar plexus chakra tensions that can be associated with symptoms include tensions about feeling controlled or not feeling free, holding oneself back from doing what one wants, feeling powerless or having an inflated sense of power, sensitivity about how one appears to others or a lack of 'ease of being', feeling that being oneself carries with it an implied threat, that it is not safe to be real and to live one's real values. Symptoms can also be the result of unexpressed or habitual anger, inner conflict about what one wants or feels, uncertainty about whether it is okay to want that, to feel that, etc. This chakra is also associated with the mental body, and tension here can be related to excessive mental activity, and control issues.

Sore Throat

A sore throat reflects unexpressed anger, and tension in the throat chakra, which is associated with expressing.

Spasms

A spasm is a sudden, involuntary contraction of a muscle or group of muscles. The site of the spasm and the chakra associated with that site reflect the tension in the consciousness that is associated with this symptom. Thus, spasms in the foot reflect root chakra tensions, with further details depending on whether it is the will foot or the emotional foot, the male foot or the female foot. Oesophageal spasms can reflect tensions in the throat chakra and/or heart chakra, etc., depending on where the discomfort is experienced. Spasms of the diaphragm reflect solar plexus tensions.

Spastic Colitis/Spastic Colon – See Irritable Bowel Syndrome

Spinal Cord

The spinal cord is associated with the nervous system and therefore the crown chakra. When the spinal cord is affected by a symptom, see the location of the symptom and the effect of the symptom. Thus, difficulty with the spinal cord at the level of the neck points to tensions about expressing (throat chakra) creating a sense of isolation (crown chakra), and if other parts of the body are affected by the symptom, see the chakra(s) associated with those parts and the effects of the symptom. If a part has been paralyzed, for example, the person has been paralyzing himself/herself and feeling isolated.

Spinal Curvature

Although the term 'spinal curvature' (or 'curvature of the spine') can refer to the normal concave and convex curvature of the spine, in clinical contexts the phrase usually refers to deviations from the expected curvature, even when that difference is a reduction in curvature. When it represents a symptom, the chakra closest to the curvature indicates the tension in the consciousness causing the curvature, and depending on whether the curvature is toward the will side or the emotional side, it indicates tensions in the will or the emotions of the individual, relative to that chakra. Thus, curvature to the will side at the level of the heart chakra reflects tensions in the person's will in the area of relationships, and the person perceiving the relationship as different from what he/she wants it to be.

Spinal Meningitis – See Meningitis

Spine

The spine is the vertebral column, also known as the backbone. Symptoms affecting the entire spine reflect root chakra tensions with money, home, job and/or mother, and insecurity as a perceptual filter. Symptoms affecting the spine in a particular location reflect tensions in the chakra closest to that location.

Spleen

The spleen is associated with the solar plexus chakra and with the person's willingness to express anger, or to 'vent their spleen'. Symptoms affecting this organ therefore reflect tensions about the person not owning their power to express anger.

Splenitis

Splenitis is an inflammation of the spleen, with enlargement of the organ and severe local pain. It is associated with the person feeling very angry about something without feeling they have the power to express the anger or do anything about the situation about which they are angry.

Spondylitis – See Ankylosing Spondylitis

Spondylolisthesis

Spondylolisthesis is a condition in which a bone (vertebra) in the spine slips out of the proper position onto the bone below it, either forward or backward. Effects can include lower back or leg pain, hamstring tightness and numbness and tingling in the legs. The chakra associated with the location of the slippage and the effect of the symptom would point to the specific tensions in the person's consciousness at the time the symptom began. When the legs are affected, it reflects tension about the root chakra parts of the person's life – money, home, job, mother – and an emotional perceptual filter of insecurity.

Spondylosis

Spondylosis describes spinal degeneration accompanied by pain, and is often used as a synonym for spinal arthritis. The chakra associated with the location of the symptom and the effect of the symptom points to the specific tensions in the person's consciousness at the time the symptom began.

Sprained Ankle

Because the legs and feet are associated with the root chakra and issues of trust, a sprained ankle on the will side of a right-handed person would reflect lack of trust in the will; the person has decided to do something but has not acted on their decision because of insecurity. On the emotional side, it would reflect emotional insecurity; the person not standing on their own two feet with regard to their emotions. Because the effect of the symptom is difficulty walking, the person has been keeping him/herself from walking away from a situation in which they are not happy, giving themselves reasons to stay in an unhappy situation. If crutches are needed, the person is soliciting support for their decisions rather than trusting themselves with those decisions.

Sprains

A sprain is an injury to the ligaments around a joint. See the part of the body and the function affected as an indicator of the inner cause. Since the joints in general are associated with the root chakra, it indicates that the function was affected by an insecurity.

Sterility

Sterility refers to not being able to have children. The capacity to produce children is associated with the sacral chakra, and from the point of view that we each create our reality, the person affected has made decisions to not have children. This reflects a wish or a decision they have made to not be a parent, or to not be a parent with the current condition in their life.

Stiff Neck

A stiff neck reflects tension in the throat chakra, and difficulty expressing. That reflects difficulty expressing emotions, or difficulty communicating. The type of stiffness could reflect further details. For example, difficulty moving the head from side to side could reflect difficulty in expressing 'No', while difficulty moving the head forward and back could reflect difficulty saying 'Yes'.

Still's Disease

Still's disease symptoms include high fever, joint inflammation and pain, muscle pain, faint salmon-coloured skin rash, swelling of the lymph glands or enlargement of the spleen and liver and inflammation of the lungs or around the heart. These symptoms reflect anger with someone close to the person. Joint inflammation and pain reflect anger about root chakra, issues which can include tension at home or with the person's mother. The person has been immobilizing him/herself with insecurity. The rash also indicates anger or possible embarrassment.

Arthritis, with joint swelling, often occurs after rash and fevers have been present for some time, again pointing to root chakra tensions, immobilizing oneself and possibly anger at one's mother.

Stings (Bee, Wasp, etc.)

An intense reaction to insect stings reflects anger. The location of the sting is not random. See the part of the body affected and the possible function affected (walking, for example) for further details.

Stomach, General

Symptoms involving the stomach reflect solar plexus tensions involving the issues of power, control, freedom and anger.

Stomach Cancer (Adenocarcinoma)

The stomach is associated with the solar plexus chakra, and the parts of the person's consciousness associated with power, control and freedom. It is also associated with the emotion of anger. Cancer represents something held in and not expressed. With stomach cancer, the person has been facing a situation involving anger or control issues, a situation that has been so unacceptable that they would rather die than continue with that situation in their life, and they have been holding on to that anger.

Stomach Ulcer

The stomach is associated with the solar plexus chakra, and ulcers reflect anger. Thus, stomach ulcers reflect tension and anger about control issues.

Strabismus – See Crossed Eyes

Strep Throat – See Tonsillitis

Stretch Marks

Stretch marks are narrow streaks or lines that develop on the surface of the skin. The areas of the body most often affected by stretch marks are the abdomen (tummy), buttocks and thighs. They develop when the skin is stretched suddenly and the middle layer of your skin (the dermis) breaks in places, allowing the deeper layers to show through. Because they are considered unsightly, and there may be sensitivities about intimate contact because of this, the symptom can reflect making oneself unattractive (in one's own eyes) because of sensitivities about intimate contact. The location is usually at the level of the sacral chakra, associated with sex, and the root chakra, associated with security or trust.

Stroke

A stroke, or cerebrovascular accident (CVA), is the rapid loss of brain function due to disturbance in the blood supply to the brain. As a result, the affected area of the brain cannot function, which might result in an inability to move one or both limbs on one side of the body, inability to understand or formulate speech or an inability to see one side of the visual field. Because the brain is affected, the symptom is associated with a closed crown chakra stimulated by tensions with father/authority, or a sense of separation from someone close.

The part(s) of the body affected reflect specific tensions in response to the event that the person responded to with stress, at the time the symptom began, and the specific decisions they made, when the effects are described from the point of view that the person created them. Thus, rather than saying that the person was paralyzed, it would be described as the person paralyzing him/herself, with further detail about the will or the emotions being paralyzed, from seeing the part of the body was affected.

Stupor

A stupor is a state of mental numbness, as that resulting from shock; a daze. The lack of responsiveness reflects crown chakra tensions and a state of isolation, as well as root chakra tensions resulting in not being present. In common usage, the word can refer to a state of intoxication in which uninhibited behaviour is apparent, with the specific behaviour reflecting specific tensions in the chakras that may have been held back in the person's everyday interactions (aggression, for example, reflecting solar plexus chakra tensions).

Stuttering

Stuttering, or stammering, is a speech disorder characterized by interruptions to speech such as hesitating, repeating sounds and words (eg. 'I-I-I-I-I can do it'), or prolonging sounds (eg. 'Where's m-m-m-my s-s-sister?'), or blocking (moments where no sounds come out when the person is trying to speak). The symptom reflects tension in the throat chakra and insecurity about communicating. Possible causes include tensions in the root chakra about not feeling safe at home, or in the crown chakra if insecure about communicating to authority/father.

Stye

A stye or sty is an infection of the eyelid, a small red bump that appears on the outside or inside of the eyelid. Because it is an irritation, it relates to feeling irritated or angry about something. If on the will eye (or male eye) it represents irritation about something contrary to what the person wants (or irritation with a male). On the emotional eye (the female eye) it represents irritation about something that touches the person emotionally (or irritation with a female).

Subarachnoid Haemorrhage

A subarachnoid haemorrhage is bleeding usually associated with aneurisms or other weakened blood vessels of the brain, which is associated with the crown chakra. Thus, it represents tensions with father/authority, or a sense of separation from someone close. The effect of the symptom, in terms of body parts or functions affected by it, points to the chakra associated with that part or function, and decisions made in response to the conditions the person reacted to.

Subdural Haematoma

In a subdural haematoma, blood collects between the layers of tissue that surround the brain, pointing to crown chakra tensions with father/authority or a sense of separation from someone close. As blood accumulates, pressure on the brain increases and may cause symptoms that can include headache, seizures and apathy, which also reflect crown chakra tensions. Other symptoms can be confusion, dizziness, lethargy or excessive drowsiness, also reflecting root chakra tensions including insecurity or fear, and weakness, nausea and vomiting, reflecting solar plexus tensions of feeling powerless to resolve an unhappy situation.

Sundown Syndrome

Sundowning, or sundown syndrome, affects some people who have Alzheimer's disease and dementia. People affected experience periods of increased confusion and agitation as the sun goes down, and sometimes through the night. People with sundown may become more forgetful, confused, delirious, agitated, anxious and/or restless, and often have trouble sleeping. They may pace the floor, wander, yell or become combative. This points to a closed crown chakra and a sense of separation or isolation, as well as possible root chakra tensions; not being present in the here and now, in addition to the sense of isolation. The behaviour (aggression, confusion, anxiety) may point to their reaction to conditions in their life at the time the symptom began, possibly missing someone no longer with them who was previously with them at night.

Sunburn

Sunburn, damage to the skin because of exposure to the sun, reflects sensitivity in the solar plexus chakra (the phrase means 'plexus of the sun') in terms of sensitivity to anger or conflict, with the part of the body affected and the chakra associated with that part giving further indication of the inner cause. Thus, sunburnt shoulders can reflect unexpressed anger, sunburnt arms reflect anger affecting one going for their goals, etc. Because the effect of the sunburn may also result in the person not wanting to be touched, that points to possible heart chakra tensions (the sense of touch is associated with the heart chakra) and crown chakra tensions (a sense of isolation or separation from someone close).

Superior Oblique Myokymia (SOM)

Superior oblique myokymia is a neurological disorder affecting vision that presents as repeated, brief episodes of movement, shimmering or shaking of the vision of one eye, a feeling of the eye trembling or vertical/tilted vision. It can result in double vision. The symptom is neurological and therefore reflects crown chakra tensions with father/authority and a sense of separation from someone close, a male if it is the male eye affected (right eye in right-handed people) or a female if it is the female eye. It also reflects the two eyes not working together and therefore a reaction to the male and female not communicating in the person's life.

Suprarenal Glands – See Adrenal Glands

Sutton's Disease – See Canker Sores

Swamp Fever

Swamp fever is an infectious disease caused by leptospira and transmitted to humans from domestic animals, and characterized by jaundice and fever, reflecting solar plexus tensions and anger. Headaches reflect crown chakra tensions and a sense of isolation. The combination points to possible anger with authority.

Swayback – See Lordosis

Swelling

Swelling, turgescence or tumefaction is enlargement of a body part or organ caused by accumulation of fluid in the tissues. It can occur through-out the body (generalized), or a specific part or organ can be affected (local-ized). It is considered one of the characteristics of inflammation along with pain, heat, redness and loss of function. Inflammation indicates anger, and the part of the body or function affected and the chakra associated with that part or function reflect the reason for the anger or the effects of the anger about what was happening in the person's life when the symptom began.

Swollen Glands

The term 'swollen glands' refers to enlargement of one or more lymph nodes. The lymph system is related to the elimination system and therefore the root chakra, and the symptom therefore relates to insecurity about something, with the part of the body affected giving further details. Thus, swollen glands in the neck refer to insecurity about expressing or communicating.

Symphysis Pubis Dysfunction (SPD) – See Pubic Bone Pain

Syncope – See Fainting

Syphilis

Syphilis is spread primarily by any sexual activity, and is considered a highly contagious disease; it is often spread through sores, reflecting anger. Any sexually transmitted disease reflects beliefs about sex being 'dirty', punishing the affected part and giving the person reasons to not have sex. People with secondary syphilis experience a rosy 'copper penny' rash typically on the palms of the hands and soles of the feet, reflecting anger keeping themselves from having what they want, and anger about root chakra issues (money, home, job). They may also experience moist warts in the groin, reflecting root chakra tensions and thus insecurity, white patches on the inside of the mouth reflecting something not communicated, swollen lymph glands (unreleased root chakra tensions or fears), fever (anger) and weight loss (not feeling nourished).

If the infection isn't treated, it may then progress to a stage characterized by severe problems with the heart (tension in relationships), brain (crown chakra tensions with authority and/or a sense of isolation) and nerves, which can result in paralysis (the person paralyzing themselves, holding themselves back, making themselves helpless in their way of thinking), blindness (feeling there is nothing to look forward to), dementia (crown chakra tensions, sense of isolation), deafness (not wanting to hear something), impotence (avoiding sex) and even death if it's not treated.

Systemic Lupus Erythematosus (SLE) – See Lupus Erythematosus

Tachycardia

Tachycardia is a fast or irregular heart rhythm, usually more than 100 beats per minute and possibly as many as 400 beats per minute. At these elevated rates, the heart is not able to efficiently pump oxygen-rich blood to your body. This can cause dizziness, light-headedness or a fluttering in the chest, which reflects tension in the heart chakra as well as the root chakra; it can reflect tension with someone close to the person's heart, at home. The person has not been allowing him/herself to feel nourished by the love around them.

Tailbone – See Coccyx

Tapeworm/Taeniasis

Tapeworms are flat segmented worms that live in the intestines of some animals and can infect humans who eat undercooked meat from those animals. Any kind of parasitic infection reflects something 'eating away' at the person's consciousness, and the effects of the symptom can point to specific areas of tension in the person's consciousness.

Tapeworms can cause signs and symptoms such as nausea (reflecting anger and control issues), weakness (solar plexus and root chakra tensions) and diarrhoea (root chakra tensions – survival, security, trust). Because tapeworms take the nourishment from the person's body, they can reflects something 'eating away' at the person that keeps them from feeling nourished by the love around them. If pork tapeworm eggs are swallowed, they can migrate to other parts of the body and cause damage to the liver (anger – tension in the solar plexus chakra), eyes (difficulty looking at something happening in the person's life), heart (heart chakra tension with someone close to the person's heart) and brain (crown chakra tension with father/authority or a sense of separation from someone close). These infections can be life-threatening if the person has been so unhappy about the situation that they would rather die than continue in that situation.

Tartar

In dentistry, calculus or tartar is a form of hardened dental plaque. It is caused by the continual accumulation of minerals from saliva on plaque on the teeth, which are associated with the root chakra. Because the eventual effect of the symptom can be gum disease and loss of teeth, it reflects root chakra tensions about money, home and job.

Tears, Lack of – See Dry Eyes

Teeth

The teeth and gums are related to the root chakra, and thus the parts of the person's life related to security – money, job, feeling safe at home – though some problems with the teeth may reflect tensions that would result in the person gritting their teeth, tightening their jaw, which is related to the solar plexus chakra. These tooth problems would then reflect anger about root chakra parts of the person's life.

Temporomandibular Joint (TMJ)

Temporomandibular disorders (TMD) occur as a result of problems with the jaw, jaw joint and surrounding facial muscles that control chewing and moving the jaw. They reflect tensions in the jaw, which is associated with the solar plexus chakra, and issues of anger, likely about root chakra parts of the person's life.

Tendonitis and Tenosynovitis

Tendonitis and tenosynovitis are types of tendon injury. Tendonitis is an irritated or inflamed tendon, pointing to anger affecting the particular function performed by that tendon. Tenosynovitis is inflammation of the tendon sheath, and reflects the same inner cause as tendonitis, but more intensely, reflecting more intense anger about the situation, to the point of the person immobilizing him/herself.

Tendons

A tendon is a fibrous connective tissue that attaches muscle to bone. Symptoms affecting the tendons affect mobility, and represent immobilizing oneself, holding oneself back from doing something because of insecurity (root chakra tensions) See the part of the body affected and the function affected for further details.

Tennis Elbow – See Epicondylalgia

Tension Myositis Syndrome (TMS)

With TMS, physical back pain is acknowledged to be the direct result of emotional factors, and not the result of physical injury to muscles or bones. See the chakra closest to the pain to understand the part of the consciousness that has been holding tension. The function or movement affected can provide further details.

Terminal Conditions

With the idea that everything begins in the consciousness, any symptom that can have death as its logical conclusion begins with a decision to die. The person is facing a situation in their life that they consider unacceptable, but they see no way out of it except to die. The person must find a way to resolve that unacceptable situation one way or another in order for them to be willing to face life.

Testicles

Though the testicles are located for functional reasons at the level of the root chakra, they are the endocrine glands associated with sex and having babies, and thus associated with and controlled by the sacral chakra. Any symptom involving the testicles reflects tension in the person's consciousness about sexual functioning or having children, though a sense of feeling castrated might also point to tensions in a relationship.

Tetanus (Lockjaw)

Tetanus causes painful tightening of the muscles, usually all over the body. It can lead to 'locking' of the jaw, which makes it difficult for the person to open their mouth or swallow. If this happens, the person could die of suffocation. The symptoms point to someone immobilizing him/herself with solar plexus energy, probably anger – and it is likely that the anger is with someone close.

Thalassaemia

Thalassaemia is a blood disorder that is considered to be inherited, passed down through families, in which the body makes an abnormal form of haemoglobin, the protein in red blood cells that carries oxygen. The symptom results in excessive destruction of red blood cells, which leads to anaemia. Symptomatically, the person is not allowing him/herself to be nourished by the love around them. While this points to a heart chakra tension, it could also be related to a closed crown chakra, in which case the person may feel they are enclosed in a shell, not feeling the love around them.

Thighs

The thighs are associated with the root chakra, and thus with the parts of the person's consciousness related to security – money, home, job and mother. When there is a symptom affecting the thighs, see what function is affected, or would be affected if the symptom were allowed to proceed, and describe it from the point of view that the person created it. Thus, if walking is affected, the person has been keeping him/herself from walking, giving him/herself reasons to remain in an unhappy situation, because of insecurity. If sexual activity is affected, the person has insecurities involving sexuality (sacral chakra tensions). Retention of fluid in the thighs points to a concentration of attention on root chakra parts of the person's life. If just one thigh is affected, see if it is the will or male thigh (right thigh in right-handed people) reflecting a question of trust in one's will or trust in a male, or the emotional or female thigh, reflecting emotional insecurity or questions of trust with a female.

Throat

Any symptom affecting the throat points to tension in the throat chakra, related to difficulty expressing or in communicating something.

Throat Chakra Tensions

The throat chakra is associated not only with the throat, but also with the shoulders, arms and hands, as well as the sense of hearing. Throat chakra tensions that can result in symptoms affecting these areas include difficulty expressing oneself and one's own truth, difficulty expressing emotions, difficulty communicating one's truth, resistance to setting goals concerning what one wants (will side) or what will make one happy (emotional side) and resistance to hearing something, or to allowing oneself to receive unconditionally.

Thrombosis

Thrombosis is a blood clot within a blood vessel. It happens when a blood clot forms and blocks a vein or an artery, obstructing or stopping the flow of blood. It points to tensions in the area of the heart chakra, tension with someone close, and the part of the body affected would point to further details about the particular decisions made by the person affected, because of this tension.

Thrush

Thrush is a yeast infection caused by a fungus called Candida albicans. Both men and women can get thrush, though it is more often associated with women. The symptoms of vaginal thrush are usually obvious and include itching and soreness around the vagina and pain during sex, pointing to tension in the sacral chakra related to sex and possibly to issues in the root chakra as well, reflecting insecurity or irritation about sex. In men it usually affects the head of the penis, causing inflammation, a smelly, lumpy discharge and pain while passing urine. It can also affect the skin, which is known as candidal skin infection, and the inside of the mouth, known as oral thrush.

Any fungal infection represents something 'eating away' at the person's consciousness, and the part of the body affected shows what it is related to. In this case, the symptom points to the person's attitudes toward sex ('Sex is dirty,' for example), and gives him/her reasons not to have sex. The person is keeping him/herself from having sex. Oral thrush can be said to be a reason for the person avoiding kissing, or avoiding participating in oral sex.

Thumbs – See Fingers

Thymus Gland

The thymus gland is associated with the immune system, and with the heart chakra, and thus with the person's perceptions of love. Symptoms that affect the immune system (AIDS, HIV, etc.) are therefore associated with tensions in the person's perceptions of love. The person feels that their lifestyle separates them from those they love. Symptoms considered autoimmune disorders can be related to tensions in the area of relationships, though the specific part of the body affected provides further details about the specific decisions made as the result of those tensions.

Thyroid

The thyroid gland is associated with the throat chakra, and therefore with the person expressing him/herself, and what is going on inside them. When this is affected by a symptom, the person has not been expressing who they really are. Either they have been showing a false persona, if the thyroid is overactive, or holding back expressing who they are, if the thyroid is under-active. See the situation they were in, and the reasons they gave themselves to not feel safe in showing who they really are.

TIA – See Transient Ischaemic Attack

Tics

Tics are rapid, repetitive, involuntary contractions of a group of muscles, usually in the face or shoulders. They represent tensions being released, tensions that keep the person from relaxing into their natural way of being – pointing to possible perceived crown chakra tensions with authority, and solar plexus chakra tensions about not experiencing ease of being. If the tic affects the will eye (right eye in right-handed people) it reflects tension about seeing what one wants, and if the emotional eye, difficulties seeing what one feels. Also see Twitch.

Tinea – See Ringworm

Tinnitus

Tinnitus is the medical term for ringing in the ears, a sound that does not have its source in the physical world. It is related to the brow chakra, associated with the non-physical element known as the inner sound. It is that deep part of the person's consciousness, their spirit, known in the Western world as their subconscious or unconscious, calling the person's attention to look inside to see if he/she is really living their truth, seeing what they really want or what they really feel, as compared to what they feel they should want or feel.

Tiredness – See Fatigue

Toes

While the toes, as part of the feet, are associated with the root chakra, specific toes have a specific meaning. Thus, on the will foot (right foot in right-handed people), the big toe is associated with the root chakra and is thus about the person trusting what they want in relation to root chakra parts of their life; the second toe is about trusting what they want in the area of the sacral chakra, food or sex or having children; the third toe is about trusting what they want in terms of solar plexus areas of their life, like freedom; the fourth toe is about trusting what they want in the area of the heart chakra; and the small toe is about trusting what they want regarding the part of their life dealing with how they express themselves or their creativity.

On the emotional foot, the big toe would reflect the person trusting their feelings about the root chakra parts of their life; the second toe, trusting their feelings about the sacral chakra parts of their life; the middle toe, trusting their feelings about the solar plexus chakra parts of their life; the fourth toe, trusting their feelings about the heart chakra parts of their life; and the little toe trusting their feelings about how they express themselves.

Tongue

The tongue is associated with different chakras, depending on the function affected, since it can be related to expressing through speech, and also sacral chakra activities and the sense of taste.

Tonsillitis (Strep Throat)

Tonsillitis, also known as strep throat, is inflammation of the tonsils most commonly caused by either viral or bacterial infection. Symptoms may include sore throat and fever, reflecting unexpressed anger at the level of the throat chakra.

Torpor

Torpor is sluggishness, dullness, stupor or a state of mental and motor inactivity with partial or total insensibility, though it is often used to describe the state of an organ such as the brain or liver when it is essentially inactive and seems to be in a state of hibernation. When applied to a person, it can relate to them lacking energy and not being totally present, reflecting root chakra tensions about money, home and job, or crown chakra tensions resulting in a state of isolation. When the word is applied to the state of an organ, see the organ and function affected for further precision.

Torticollis

Torticollis, also known as 'wry neck', is a painful disorder of the muscles in the neck. Different types of torticollis may have different symptoms. The faces of some children with fixed torticollis may look unbalanced or flattened (plagiocephaly). The muscle contractions involved in cervical dystonia can cause the head to twist in a variety of directions. There is a limited range of motion of the head, headache, head tremor and neck pain. The symptom reflects tension in the throat chakra and crown chakra, pointing to difficulty expressing, and tensions with authority/father.

Tourette's Syndrome

Tourette's syndrome (TS) is a neurological disorder characterized by repetitive, involuntary movements and vocalizations called tics, including motor movements that result in self-harm such as punching oneself in the face or vocal tics including uttering socially inappropriate words such as swearing, or repeating the words or phrases of others. As a neurological symptom it reflects crown chakra tensions, and the person holding themselves back from expressing themselves naturally for concerns of how it may seem for authority, as well as experiencing a sense of isolation. The tensions of holding themselves back are released during the episodes of the syndrome, along with anger at themselves as a form of punishment for having the wish to express what is considered socially unacceptable.

Toxaemia

Toxaemia is a what physicians refer to as pregnancy-induced hypertension. Some of the characteristics include high blood pressure and fluid retention. Complications can include jaundice or yellowing of the eyes and skin, severe headaches, excessive weight gain associated with fluid retention especially in the face and hands or ankles, blurred vision and easy bleeding or bruising. Severe cases can cause restriction of blood flow to the placenta, causing harm to the foetus, seizures in the mother, coma or even death of either the mother or the foetus. The symptoms point to heart chakra tensions with someone close, solar plexus tensions and strong anger and crown chakra tensions and a sense of separation or isolation, as well as emotional sensitivity and possible ambivalence about being pregnant at that time, possibly due to tensions with the partner.

Toxoplasmosis

Toxoplasmosis symptoms include mild flu-like symptoms, such as high temperature, sore throat and aching muscles, reflecting anger and tensions in the solar plexus chakra, associated with a perceived lack of power in the current situation in the person's life.

Congenital toxoplasmosis occurs when a woman becomes infected during pregnancy and passes the infection on to her unborn baby. This can result in the baby developing serious health problems such as blindness and brain damage, reflecting a reaction to not feeling the contact with its parents. This raises questions about tensions between the parents and possible ambivalence about having the child at that time.

Transient Ischaemic Attack (TIA)

A transient ischaemic attack (TIA) or 'mini stroke' is caused by a temporary disruption in the blood supply to part of the brain, resulting in a lack of oxygen to the brain. The symptoms are similar to those of a stroke, such as speech and visual disturbance and numbness or weakness in the arms and legs. Because the brain is associated with the crown chakra, the tensions in the consciousness reflect tensions with father or authority, or a sense of separation from someone close. See the parts of the body affected for further details of decisions made at that time. If the face is affected, having fallen on one side, the person may be unable to smile, or their mouth or eye may have dropped, and that specific symptom points to brow chakra tensions and a sense of having felt 'slapped in the face', figuratively, in a way that they responded to by paralyzing themselves on either the will side or the emotional side.

Tremors

Tremors are unintentional trembling or shaking movements in one or more parts of the body. Most tremors occur in the hands but one can also have arm, head, face, vocal cord, trunk and leg tremors. Because tremors are related to nerve impulses to the affected part, they can be related to crown chakra tensions with authority. See the part affected for further details about the person's response to those tensions and where they may have been feeling ambivalence about their actions.

Trigeminal Nerves

The trigeminal nerves are associated with sensation in the face and certain motor functions such as chewing. When these nerves are affected, and there is a burning sensation to the side of the face, it is associated with the brow chakra and the person having felt deeply insulted – 'slapped in the face' – on either the will side or the emotional side.

Trochanteritis

Trochanteritis is also known as trochanteric bursitis and is a type of hip bursitis, an inflammation of the bursa located near the greater trochanter of the femur.

As an inflammation, it represents anger, and being in the hip, it points to the root chakra parts of the person's life – money, home, job – and issues of insecurity or mistrust. On the male or will side (right side in right-handed people) it reflects issues of trust with a man, or trusting one's will in relation to what was happening in the person's life at the time the symptom began, and on the female or emotional side it represents questions of trust with a female or the person not feeling supported emotionally. See Bursitis.

Tubal Pregnancy – See Ectopic Pregnancy

Tuberculosis (TB)

Tuberculosis is an infection, primarily in the lungs (a pneumonia). The most common symptoms of TB are fatigue (root chakra tensions, possibly at home), fever (anger, solar plexus chakra tensions), weight loss (possibly root chakra, not feeling nourished by the love at home), coughing (heart chakra, anger with someone close) and night sweats (root chakra – elimination system – and solar plexus tensions). The symptoms point to heart chakra tensions in the person's perceptions of love, and anger issues with someone close, possibly at home.

Tuberculous Spondylitis – See Pott's Disease

Tumours

Tumours represent something held in and not expressed, and the location of the tumour and the function that was affected points to what it is that has not been expressed, depending on the chakra involved with that part or with the function affected. As an example, lung cancer affects the person's ability to breathe; and since the heart chakra is associated with the element of air, it can be said that a person's relationship with air is a reflection of their relationship with love. Thus, difficulty breathing can be related to heart chakra tensions and the person's willingness to let in the love (inhale) or express it (exhale) because of tensions in the person's consciousness with someone close when the symptom began.

Malignant (life-threatening) tumours are symptomatically similar to benign tumours, but since they are life-threatening, they represent tensions that have been accompanied by the decision to die. The person affected does not want to face life with the unacceptable situation they reacted to, so then they must find a resolution to that situation.

Twitch (Benign Fasciculation Syndrome)

Benign fasciculation syndrome (twitching) is a neurological disorder characterized by twitching of various voluntary muscles in the body. The twitching can occur in any voluntary muscle group but is most common in the eyelids, arms, legs and feet.

Because it is a neurological problem (crown chakra – relationship with authority) affecting the muscles (solar plexus chakra – issues of control), it can be seen as a conflict between the person's will and authority. The person is nervous about issues with authority and about expressing him/herself naturally. See the part of the body affected for more detail.

If the twitching is in the eyelid, it can be seen as the person having difficulty looking at some issue. If it is the will eye (the right eye in right-handed individuals) it can reflect being nervous about what one wants, and if it is the emotional eye (the left eye in right-handed individuals), an emotional reaction to issues with authority.

Typhoid Fever

Typhoid fever, also known as enteric fever, is a potentially fatal illness. The classic presentation includes fever, malaise, diffuse abdominal pain and constipation. Symptoms may include intestinal haemorrhage, bowel perforation and death within one month of onset. It reflects solar plexus tensions of anger and strong root chakra symptoms of not feeling safe at home.

Ulcerated Cornea

A corneal ulcer is an open sore on the cornea, the thin clear structure overlying the iris, which is the coloured part of your eye. Depending on whether it is the male eye (right eye in right-handed people) or the female eye, it reflects anger with either a male or a female at the time the symptom began. See Cornea.

Ulcerative Colitis

Ulcerative colitis is a disease that causes inflammation and sores (ulcers) in the lining of the large intestine (colon). The symptoms point to anger about the root chakra parts of the person's life at the time the symptom began. The disease can also cause other problems, such as joint pain, also reflecting root chakra tensions, liver disease, reflecting anger and solar plexus chakra tensions, and eye problems, also reflecting solar plexus chakra tensions and difficulty looking at a situation the person is unhappy about.

Ulcers

Ulcers as a symptom reflect anger, and the part of the body affected reflects more details. Stomach ulcers, for example, reflect anger about issues of control or freedom.

Uraemia

Uraemic syndrome (uraemia) is a serious complication of chronic kidney disease and acute renal failure. It reflects the person feeling helpless to change an unhappy situation, and making themselves helpless in their way of thinking ('I can't...'). It may affect any part of the body and can cause nausea and vomiting, reflecting solar plexus tensions, anger and feeling that they are out of control; weight loss that reflects the person not feeling nourished; and changes in mental status, such as confusion, reduced awareness, agitation, psychosis, seizures and coma – reflecting root chakra tensions and insecurity as well as not being present in the here and now, as well as crown chakra tensions with father/authority and a sense of separation from someone, isolation.

Heart problems, such as an irregular heartbeat, inflammation of and excess fluid in the sac that surrounds the heart (pericarditis), increased pressure on the heart and shortness of breath, all point to heart chakra tensions with someone close and difficulty letting in the love.

Ureteritis

Ureteritis refers to a medical condition of the ureter that involves inflammation. The ureters are tubes made of smooth muscle fibres that propel urine from the kidneys to the urinary bladder. The condition reflects anger about the root chakra parts of one's life – money, home, job, mother. Because it can be due to the passing of a kidney stone and therefore may reflect kidney symptoms as well, it also reflects a sense of helplessness or powerlessness about an unhappy situation

Urethritis

Urethritis is inflammation of the urethra, the tube that connects the urinary bladder to the outside of the body and includes the opening at the end of the penis. Symptoms affecting this part reflect tensions in the root chakra, and thus insecurity about something, and because sexual functions may also be affected, tensions in the sacral chakra as well, which is associated with sex. Thus, the insecurities may also be about sexual issues.

Urinary System

The urinary system is part of the elimination system, and thus associated with the root chakra, and the root chakra parts of the person's life – money, home, job, mother. Symptoms affecting the urinary system thus reflect insecurity and tensions in these areas.

Urticaria – See Hives

Uterus, General

The uterus is a hollow muscular organ located in the female pelvis. The main function of the uterus is to nourish the developing foetus prior to birth. In general, it is associated with the sacral chakra and having children. Symptoms here may reflect tensions in this area, though because of its physical location at the level of the root chakra, certain symptoms involving the uterus may also reflect lack of trust with a specific male or with men more generally.

Uterus Fibroma (Uterine Fibroids)

Uterine fibroids are lumps, generically and symptomatically considered as tumours, which grow on the uterus. They represent something held in and not expressed, and the possible logical conclusion of the symptom may be to remove the uterus, thus making it unlikely that the woman will have a child. The fibroids thus reflect ambivalence about having a child at the time the symptom developed, or questions of trust with a man.

Vaginal Yeast Infections

A yeast infection causes itching or soreness in the vagina and sometimes causes pain or burning when urinating or having sex. These symptoms reflect tensions in the root chakra (insecurity) and sacral chakra. Irritation reflects anger. Some women also have a thick, clumpy, white discharge that has no odour and looks a little like cottage cheese. The effect of the symptom would be to discourage sexual activity. Thus, the person is keeping herself from having sex – wanting sex but giving herself reasons not to do so, perhaps with the feeling that sex is dirty.

Vaginitis

Vaginitis is an inflammation of the vagina. It can result in discharge, itching and pain, and is often associated with an irritation or infection of the vulva. The symptoms reflect irritation (anger) in the area of sexuality, and insecurity in this area, because of its location at the level of the root chakra. The effect of the symptom would be to discourage sexual activity. Thus, the person is keeping herself from having sex – wanting sex but giving herself reasons not to do so, because of insecurity or anger.

Varicella Zoster Virus (VZV) – See Shingles

Varicoceles

Varicoceles are enlarged varicose veins that occur in the scrotum and are associated with infertility, and which may cause pain and atrophy of the testicles. This reflects tension in the sacral chakra, associated with sexuality and the person's ability to have children. The person affected is giving himself reasons for not having children. Varicoceles are said to occur most often in the left testicle, reflecting emotional conflicts about sex or having children, where what the person wants may be in conflict with certain values. Pain in the area also gives the person affected reasons for not having sex. The symptoms may also point to a possible sense of having felt castrated by a partner.

Varicose Veins

Varicose veins are twisted, enlarged veins near the surface of the skin. They most commonly develop in the legs and ankles. Because the flow of blood is associated with the heart chakra, and the location of the symptom is at the level of the root chakra, the symptoms reflect tension about the circulation of love with the mother, or the circulation of love at home. If walking is affected, the person has been giving him/herself reasons to stay in a difficult situation, rather than walking away.

Variola – See Smallpox

Vasovagal Attack (Fainting)

A vasovagal attack happens because blood pressure drops, reducing circulation to the brain and causing loss of consciousness. The tracking on the physical level points to heart chakra tensions (circulation of blood) and crown chakra tensions (brain), including a sense of isolation – though the effect is of the person experiencing insecurity or fear and leaving their body, and therefore disconnecting at the level of the root chakra. Someone predisposed to fainting or going out of their body is therefore experiencing tension in the root chakra parts of their life (likely tensions at home or with their mother) and insecurity or fear as a perceptual filter.

Venereal Disease

A venereal disease is a disease that is contracted and transmitted by sexual contact, reflecting tensions in the sacral chakra, mixed feelings about sex and possible beliefs that sex is an unhealthy activity. The particular effect of the symptom can point to further details of the tensions in the consciousness of the person affected. For example, AIDS is considered a sexually transmitted disease (STD), though symptomatically it is related to the heart chakra and thus the person's perceptions of love, the person feeling that their sexual lifestyle separates them from those they love. While hepatitis may be transmitted sexually, it is a liver disorder and therefore associated with the solar plexus chakra and anger, as well as a sense of isolation, pointing to crown chakra tensions.

Vertigo

Vertigo is dizziness, pointing to root chakra tensions and a sense of insecurity or fear, and not feeling grounded. It is often associated with nausea and vomiting, a sense of things going out of control, as well as a balance disorder, causing difficulties standing or walking and the person going out of their body.

Viral Hepatitis

Viral hepatitis is liver inflammation due to a viral infection. It represents anger and isolation, and thus tension in the solar plexus and crown chakras.

Vision Problems, General

In general, vision problems represent solar plexus tensions and difficulty in dealing with a certain situation in the person's life at the time the symptom began. The type of vision difficulty reflects the individual decisions the person made in response to the conditions in their life at the time the symptom began. See Eyes.

Vitiligo

Vitiligo is a condition that causes depigmentation of sections of skin. Because the pigment and sensitivity to light is associated with the crown chakra, and the effect can be experienced as 'creating' a sense of isolation/separation from others, the symptom is related to crown chakra tensions with the father/authority, or having felt separation from someone close. When there is also a sensitivity to the sun associated with this condition, it reflects sensitivity to solar plexus chakra issues – sensitivity about confrontation/conflict /control.

Voice

If there is a symptom affecting the voice, there is tension in the throat chakra and the person has been keeping him/herself from expressing, avoiding communicating, possibly about something specific and sensitive.

Vomit

Vomiting is a release of tension from the solar plexus chakra, letting go of control or a sense of things going out of control.

Vulva

The vulva is the external genital organ of the female. Symptoms affecting this part reflect tensions in the area of sexuality, since the effect can be to discourage sexual contact. Because the location is also at the level of the root chakra, root chakra tensions and insecurity (possibly about sex) are additional considerations.

Vulvodynia

Vulvodynia is persistent, unexplained pain in the vulva. It reflects tensions in the area of sexuality, since the effect can be to discourage sexual contact. Because the location is at the level of the root chakra, root chakra tensions and insecurity (possibly about sex) are additional considerations.

Walking Problems

Described from the point of view that we each create our reality, difficulty walking represents the person keeping him/herself from walking – giving oneself reasons to stay in an unhappy situation. Because the symptom also reflects tension in the root chakra, it points to insecurity as the reason for the person not 'walking away.'

Wall Eyes

When the two eyes are not working together, it can be described as the male eye and the female eye not working together, and this reflects the person's reaction to his/her parents representing a non-harmonious polarity. In such a case, the person could have difficulty being open to both energies at the same time, and the two sides of the brain would not be working together. Other symptoms of this same situation could be dyslexia or symptoms always affecting one side of the body and not the other.

Warthin's Tumour

Warthin's tumour is most commonly found in the parotid gland, the salivary gland. As a tumour, it represents something held in and not expressed. The location might affect the larynx (voice box), reflecting unexpressed anger, or it might affect the lymph glands, reflecting insecurity about expressing, or anger about the root chakra parts of the person's life related to security at the time the symptom began. See Salivary Glands.

Warts

Warts are small, rough non-cancerous lumps. They often develop on the skin of the hands and feet and usually disappear on their own. The inner cause is indicated by the part of the body and function affected. Thus, on the feet they represent root chakra tensions, particularly if they affect walking or standing; the foot affected would reflect tensions on the will side or emotional side and thus, insecurities involving either the will or the emotions. Genital warts reflect sensitivities in the area of sexuality, and possible beliefs about sex being 'dirty.' Warts on the hands can represent sensitivities about the person allowing him/herself to have fulfilment of something they have asked for, though it might also create sensitivities about touching others, and thus other social reasons.

Wasp Stings – See Stings

Water Retention – See Oedema

Weakness

Weakness is a symptom represented, medically, by a number of different conditions, including lack of muscle strength, dizziness or fatigue, and thus represents tension in the solar plexus and not owning one's power, or root chakra tensions and insecurities about the root chakra parts of the person's life – money, home, job and/or mother.

Whitlow

A Whitlow is a painful infection on the fingers caused by the herpes simplex virus. It is also known as herpetic Whitlow. Whitlow may be accompanied by more general symptoms, such as fever, enlarged lymph nodes or red streaking on the hands or arms. The symptom reflects anger related to having a particular issue as a goal, with the anger preventing the person from achieving that goal. See the finger affected for further details. Also see Fingers.

Whooping Cough

Whooping cough is a bacterial infection of the lungs and airways, pointing to heart chakra tensions, and anger at someone close. Because it is considered highly contagious, it also reflects crown chakra tensions and a sense of isolation, or separation from someone close.

The condition usually begins with a persistent dry and irritating cough that progresses to intense bouts of coughing. Because it is related to the heart chakra and the element of air, one's relationship with air reflects one's relationship with love, and here, the air is being pushed away; the individual affected is pushing away someone's love. Other symptoms include a runny nose, reflecting root chakra tensions and insecurity, and raised temperature and vomiting after coughing, reflecting anger and solar plexus tensions. When it is an infant who is affected, it is interesting to see how they may have felt separated from one or both parents at the time the symptom began.

Wisdom Tooth (Impacted)

Wisdom teeth, or third molars, are the last teeth to develop and appear in your mouth. When a tooth is unable to fully enter the mouth because there is not enough room, it is said to be 'impacted.' If left in the mouth, impacted wisdom teeth may damage neighbouring teeth, or become infected, and may lead to possible systemic infections and illnesses that affect the heart, kidneys and other organs. The teeth are related to the root chakra, and symptoms involving the teeth therefore reflect root chakra tensions about money, home, work or mother. In the rare cases where the heart may be affected, that would reflect heart chakra tensions with someone close at home, and kidney difficulties reflect the person feeling helpless to change an unhappy situation.

Womb – See Uterus

Wrist

The wrist is associated with the throat chakra, and the person's willingness or ability to allow him/herself to have something they have previously asked for from the universe. On the will side, it would reflect difficulty letting him/herself have what they want, and on the emotional side, difficulty with or resistance to having what would make them happy.

Wry Neck – See Torticollis

Xanthelasmas

Xanthelasmas are small yellow deposits seen on the eyelid and may be related to cirrhosis, a symptom affecting the liver and therefore reflecting anger and solar plexus tensions. This symptom is said to possibly indicate elevated cholesterol levels and may therefore point to anger with someone close to the person's heart – a partner, parent, sibling or child. See whether it is the male eye or the female eye affected. If the effect of the symptom, if allowed to proceed to its logical conclusion, would be to close the eye, it could represent not seeing the male, or not seeing the female; tensions with men or women in the person's life.

Yeast Infections (Vaginal)

The effects of a yeast infection can include itching and irritation, pointing to the person feeling irritated in the area of the root chakra, affecting their sexuality. Thus, it reflects insecurity about sexuality, and a feeling that somehow, sex is dirty. Because it is a fungal infection, it represents something 'eating away' at the person's sense of security in the area of sexuality.

Zona – See Shingles

Index

About the Author

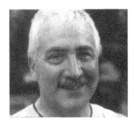

Martin Brofman dedicated his life to providing tools for healing and transformation, for self-development and spiritual awakening. He created the Body Mirror System of Healing and A Vision Workshop, as the result of his research into the body/mind connection, and from what he learned healing himself of terminal cancer in 1975. He worked with and taught these methods around the world until 2014 when he passed away.

Martin is the author of *Anything Can Be Healed* and *Improve Your Vision*, two books that have been translated into and published in more than twenty languages. He dedicated the last two years of his life to the writing of this, his final book. As founder and director of the Brofman Foundation for the Advancement of Healing, Martin was dedicated to promoting healing in the world, as well as coordinating the activities of the various instructors teaching his methods. He believed and worked with the idea that we are all healers, and that anything can be healed. His teachings played a role in many people's lives and the quality of his love touched some very deeply.

His wife, Annick Brofman, and other instructors trained by Martin are continuing his work, teaching classes successfully around the world. The Brofman Foundation for the Advancement of Healing in Switzerland, now directed by Annick, continues to be involved in gathering information and advancing healing as a process in the world.

For information (worldwide classes, posters, meditation) contact Annick Brofman at angel@healer.ch or visit https://brofman-foundation.org

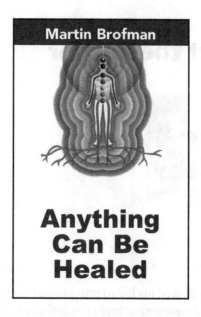

Martin Brofman

Anything Can Be Healed

Providing powerful healing methods, techniques,
and tools anyone can use, Martin Brofman reveals
how the physical body and its tensions and
symptoms are a mirror of the consciousness within.
He explains how to trace physical symptoms to
their emotional or mental causes and work
with them in his Body Mirror System.

ISBN 9781844090167

Chakra Reference Charts

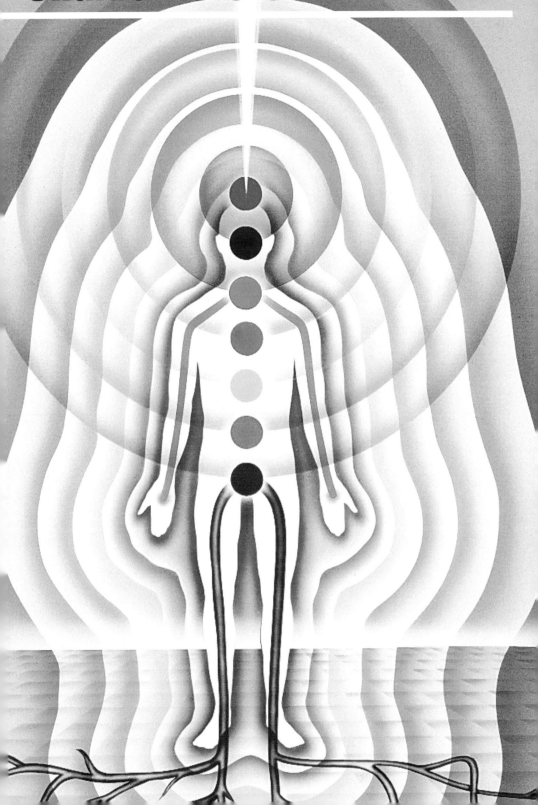

THE CHAKRAS

STRUCTURE

Yang
Male
Will
Acting

CAUSAL BODY
BUDDHIC (NIRVANIC) BODY
ETHERIC BODY
ASTRAL BODY
MENTAL BODY
EMOTIONAL BODY
PHYSICAL BODY

Vibrations	**Nerves**	System
Musical Notes	Glands	**Elements**
Violet	**Brain**	Nervous System
B Si	Pineal	**Inner Light**
Indigo	**Carotid Plexus**	Growth, Endocrine System
A La	Pituitary	**Inner Sound**
Blue	**Cervical Plexus**	Metabolism
G Sol	Thyroïd	**Ether**
Green	**Cardiac Plexus**	Respiration, Circulation, Immune System
F FA	Thymus	**Air**
Yellow	**Solar Plexus**	Skin, Muscles, Digestive System
E Mi	Pancreas	**Fire**
Orange	**Lombar Plexus**	Assimilation and Reproduction
D Re	Gonads	**Water**
Red	**Sacral Plexus**	Skeleton, Lymph, Elimination System
C Do	Adrenals	**Earth**

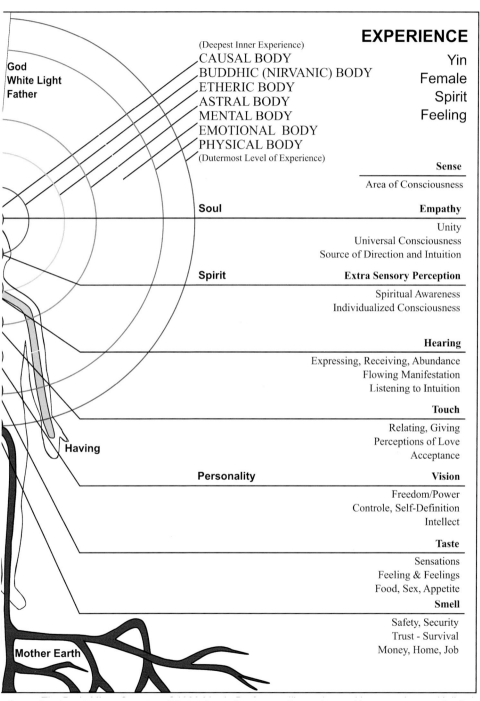

EXPERIENCE

God
White Light
Father

(Deepest Inner Experience)
CAUSAL BODY
BUDDHIC (NIRVANIC) BODY
ETHERIC BODY
ASTRAL BODY
MENTAL BODY
EMOTIONAL BODY
PHYSICAL BODY
(Outermost Level of Experience)

Yin
Female
Spirit
Feeling

Sense

Area of Consciousness

Soul   **Empathy**

Unity
Universal Consciousness
Source of Direction and Intuition

Spirit   **Extra Sensory Perception**

Spiritual Awareness
Individualized Consciousness

Hearing

Expressing, Receiving, Abundance
Flowing Manifestation
Listening to Intuition

Touch

Relating, Giving
Perceptions of Love
Acceptance

Having

Personality   **Vision**

Freedom/Power
Controle, Self-Definition
Intellect

Taste

Sensations
Feeling & Feelings
Food, Sex, Appetite

Smell

Safety, Security
Trust - Survival
Money, Home, Job

Mother Earth

The Body Mirror System   © 1988 Martin Brofman   Illustration and layout: Jørgen Højland

Tensions in the Human Energy Field

Chakras	Parts of the Body	Parts of the Consciousness	Tensions in Chakra
Crown	Brain, head, hair, nervous system, pineal gland.	Unity versus isolation, sense of direction, connection with father, authority.	Tensions could be experienced as conflict with authority and/or feeling isolated or separated from someone close. Often, the person's relationship with their father establishes the pattern for their relationship with authority and with their god(s).
Brow	Forehead, pituitary gland, trigeminal nerves, carotid plexus.	Spirit (unconscious, subconscious), subtle senses (ESP like clairvoyance, clairaudience etc.).	Tensions could be experienced as not listening to one's inner voice, or not feeling at ease with one's body, or having felt a deep conflict about not being seen for who one is..
Throat	Throat, arms, wrists, hands, fingers, thyroid gland, ears, sense of hearing.	Expressing, receiving, communicating, setting goals.	Tensions could be experienced as difficulty communicating or expressing oneself, or difficulty expressing emotions.
Heart	Heart, blood circulatory system, lungs, thymus gland, immune system. Sense of touch.	Perceptions of love, the area of relationships, people close to your heart, like partners, parents, siblings, children.	Tensions reflect conflict or disappointment with someone close, not feeling loved or tensions about being in a relationship (or not being in one).
Solar plexus	All organs located mid-body, as well as skin, muscles, jaw. Eyes. Sense of sight	Power, control, freedom. Ease of being.	Tension can be related to anger or control issues, or tension about freedom, or how the person feels about how they are seen by others.
Sacral	Gonads, sense of taste. Sexual organs and glands. Tongue.	Relationship with food, sex and having children.	Tensions can be related to tension or ambivalence about sex or having children, or the person not listening to what their body is asking for in terms of food or sex.
Root	Legs, elimination system, skeletal system, lymph system, adrenal glands. Sense of smell. Nose. Teeth and gums.	Security, survival, trust; the parts of your life having to do with safety	Tensions can be experienced as fear, insecurity or mistrust, and can be related to tensions about the home, about money or work, difficulty letting in love from one's mother. Often, a person's relationship with their mother sets the pattern for their relationship with everything that represents security.